Food

Wolfson College Lectures

Food	Edited by Barbara Harriss-White and Sir Raymond Hoffenberg
The Science of New Materials	Edited by Andrew Briggs
The Simulation of Human Intelligence	Edited by Donald Broadbent
Memory	Edited by Thomas Butler
Revolution and Counter-Revolution	Edited by Ellen Rice

Food

Multidisciplinary Perspectives

Edited by

Barbara Harriss-White

and

Sir Raymond Hoffenberg

BLACKWELL
Oxford UK & Cambridge USA

First published 1994

Blackwell Publishers
108 Cowley Road
Oxford OX4 1JF
UK

238 Main Street
Cambridge, Massachusetts 02142
USA

British Library Cataloguing in Publication Data
A CIP catalogue record for this book is available from the British Library.

Library of Congress Cataloging-in-Publication Data
Food: multidisciplinary perspectives / edited by Barbara Harriss-White
and Sir Raymond Hoffenberg.
p. cm. — (Wolfson College lectures; 1992)
Includes bibliographical references and index.
ISBN 0–631–18828–2 (alk. paper)
1. Food supply—Government policy. 2. Nutrition policy. 3. Human rights.
I. Harriss-White, Barbara II. Hoffenberg, R. (Raymond) III. Series.
HD9000.6.F576 1994
363.8—dc20 93–30500
CIP

Typeset in 10 on 11½ pt Bembo
by Graphicraft Typesetting Ltd., Hong Kong
Printed in Great Britain by Hartnolls Ltd., Bodmin

This book is printed on acid-free paper

Contents

Figures

Tables

Contributors

Professor Philip Alston
Centre for International and Public Law, Australian National University, Canberra ACT 2601, Australia

Mr Ross Buckland
Unigate plc, Unigate House, Wood Lane, London

Professor Harriet Friedmann
Department of Sociology, University of Toronto, Ontario, Canada

Professor John Garrow
St Bartholomew's Hospital, London

Dr Barbara Harriss-White
Wolfson College, Oxford

Professor Sir Raymond Hoffenberg
Wolfson College, Oxford

Professor W. P. T. James
Rowett Research Institute, Bucksburn, Aberdeen

Professor Michael Lipton
Institute of Development Studies,
University of Sussex, Brighton

Professor S. W. Mintz
Department of Anthropology, Johns Hopkins University, Baltimore, Maryland 21218 USA

Professor Onora O'Neill
Newnham College, Cambridge

Professor P. R. Payne
Centre for Human Nutrition, London School of Hygiene and Tropical Medicine, Keppel Street, London

Professor A. S. Truswell
Human Nutrition Unit, Department of Biochemistry, University of Sydney NSW 2006, Australia

Dr A. Whitehead
School of Social Sciences, University of Sussex, Brighton

Acknowledgements

The core of this book comprised the Wolfson College Lectures of 1992. The editors express deep gratitude to the original crew of eight lecturers, to Stewart Truswell, Onora O'Neill and Philip Alston who joined the project at a later stage, and to Steve Smith and Brigitte Lee at Blackwell Publishers. We gratefully acknowledge the United Nations University, Tokyo and Westview Press respectively for permission to publish the following papers: Alston, P. (1984) 'International law and the human right to food', in A. Eide, W. B. Eide, S. Goonatilake, J. Gusson and Omawale (eds) *Food as a Human Right*, pp. 162–74, copyright © (1984) by the United Nations University, all rights reserved; and O'Neill, O. (1988) 'Hunger, needs, and rights', in S. Luper-Fry (ed.) *Problems of International Justice*, pp. 67–83. Last, but not least, our thanks go to the staff of Wolfson College, Oxford, particularly to Janet Walker, without all of whose unstinting help neither the lecture series, the convivial evenings following the discussion, nor this book would have been possible. We dedicate this volume to the memory of Erica Wheeler, former Head of the Centre of Human Nutrition at the London School of Hygiene and Tropical Medicine and well known to most of our contributors, who died in 1992.

why diet + food is important.

1

Introduction

Barbara Harriss-White

Only the most obdurate of neoclassical economists for whom one commodity is much like another would deny the special nature of food. Food is special in many respects. It is the foundation, along with water, of our survival. It is both a basic need and a basic pleasure. As Audrey Richards explains: 'nutrition is more fundamental than sex. In the life of an individual it is the primary recurrent want while in the wider sphere of society it determines . . . the nature of social groups and the form their activities take'.[1] Food is a carefully chosen and classified means of social communication and the object of a richly expressive and varied aesthetic. Its production and distribution is a provider of work and livelihoods and the source of legitimacy to governments. It is an important building block of international relations. It is thus also a subject of conflict within the household, between social groups, between nations. Food excludes. It is a source of disease and of discontent. Its production is one reason for environmental transformation and sometimes for its degradation and destruction. Food may be a cause of dependence and subordination. It is a tool of war. By examining the role played by food we come to understand much that is basic to human society as a whole.

Yet in treating food as special we run some risks. We isolate this subject from other aspects of social life and in so doing we may exaggerate our capacity to manipulate society in ways which might lead to better distributions. We emphasize one aspect of rural economies increasingly dependent for survival on the diversification of their activity bases. We wrench food from its context of other global commodities (such as oil) on its interaction with which the food economy depends. We label as 'for humans' crops which may also be heading 'for animals', or more starkly 'for the manufacture of industrial alcohol', the multiple destinations of which may affect the supply of food itself. There is no easy boundary defined by food.

For 1992, Wolfson College, Oxford, chose this subject for its public lecture series with two purposes over and above Kipling's 'satiable curtiosity'. One was to forge connections between the applied sciences of medicine, nutrition and food science on the one hand, and economics, politics and anthropology on the other. The second aim was to review the scope of the contributions of these disciplines to our understanding of the many roles played by food in the obstinately modernizing world. This collection covers both advanced, OECD societies and underdeveloped, Third World ones. Our contributors have also spontaneously risen to a challenge hardly visible on the original agenda, and have suggested social solutions to some of the many problems they have identified and which were taken up in discussion. For that reason, and also for the sake of completeness, legal and ethical arguments for distributive justice have been added to this interdisciplinary collection.

Links between disciplines are manifest at two levels. First, there is a surprising convergence of method. This may tell us more about the strait-jacket of a public lecture than about scientific methodologies. More often than not, our contributors have exposed case study and/or experimental evidence to treatments which are comparativist, critical and at times polemical. Second, the structure of the series of lectures, and of the chapters here, reveals disciplines at work at a continuum of scales from that of metabolic pathways within the body, and from individual nutrients, via the scale of the person as a sentient, social (and at times sick) being, through to industries, economies, global politics, global laws and globally relevant ideas of rights and obligations.

In this introduction, a different order for our discussion of food enables us to contextualize issues raised by the lectures and to point to some of the most important areas of controversy. We shall consider production, distribution and consumption before confronting the breakdown of food systems and facing the pressure to prescribe.

The Production of Food

The United Nations' Food and Agriculture Organization (FAO) has reckoned that less than half the world's potential arable land is under cultivation. Using advanced agricultural technology it would be possible to produce food to sustain 33 billion people – seven times the present world population – and our current population could be fed on a simple but adequate diet of vegetarian and range-based animal products by systems of production in which fertilizer, agrochemicals and high-yielding varieties did not have to be used. Even though global food productivity gains are slackening or have plateaued, if there are problems in the production of food, as our book suggests, they are not of technical limitation.

The first food production problem is one of maldistribution. It is easier to perceive that cropping potential is unevenly spread, than to understand how the natural environment has come to be profoundly modified by social actions. Production is affected by uneven distribution not just of land quality but of people's rights to land and to water, unequal access to labour, credit and tools, inequalities in the control over the results of food production and over the labour of the different genders. These spatial, environmental and social maldistributions in production set conditions for specialization, technical change and trade. Comparative advantage and disadvantage are thus socially constructed. At the same time, skewed distributions of the factors of production may hinder production and create the preconditions for unequal levels of consumption.

The second problem concerns the transformation of the ways in which food production is organized. Throughout the food-producing world, whether in Iowa or Chengdu, market exchange is permeating systems of production. So far with few exceptions, market exchange has succeeded less in removing and more in perpetuating the maldistributions listed above. As Lipton observes in chapter 8 of this volume, poverty and production are concentrated in food-growing areas. Indifferent production and low consumption are frequently associated with poverty – especially when the poor are not only peasant producers but are also assetless agricultural labourers and especially when these labourers are women. In one region of India, for a vivid illustration, female labourers have been found to be paid at the end of the working day in kind rather than cash, but with raw cotton. These food producers are then compelled into multiple market transactions to acquire food – in this case the markets for labour, for cotton, for money and, finally, for the millet needed for their survival.

A third set of production problems involves the impact of technical changes in food production, the first generation of which took the form of transfers of technology – from the American Midwest to Mexico to India in the case of wheat and maize; and from the Philippines to South and South-East Asia and to West Africa in the case of rice. Originally funded by American Foundations through the profits of petrochemicals, automobile and food industries, and later multilateralized, a network of 17 food research institutes has been developed for key agro-ecological regions in order to rectify the imbalance in research resource allocation (though such food research still absorbs under 1 per cent of total resources for agricultural research and the latter are less than 1 per cent of global defence research expenditure). While most agricultural research is demand-driven and tends to respond to the relative scarcities of resources used for food production, this publicly funded food research effort is driven by the suppliers of funds to fulfil mandates to develop technologies for a constituency which is (in terms of development policy) relatively inarticulate and politically weak. So it is hardly surprising that the early high-yielding varieties of food staples represented transfers of technology developed for conditions of relative land and labour scarcity and of capital abundance often inappropriate to the physical and social environments to which they were transferred.

The new technology wended its way through societies operating not only on the profit-maximizing logic of *femina economica* but also on a rich variety of other principles: of risk aversion; of fixed production or income goals; of collective obligations to redistribute wealth and guarantee livelihoods; of effort driven by the needs of dependents; of coercive subordination. Nevertheless, the first generation of high-yielding varieties were associated with a very important trebling of rice output in Asia, roughly one-third due to the yield potential of the seeds themselves, one-third due to the application of fertilizer and one-third due to controlled water availability.[2] Early reports of the economic impact of this technical transformation in Asia pointed, however, to its spatial and social patchiness, to its association with increasing income inequality (whether or not the poor actually grew poorer), to net labour displacement, to increasing tenurial insecurity and to undeveloped supporting institutions, for example those providing information and marketing. There is now no doubt that small-scale producers lagged behind large ones in adopting new technology, though whether this set the poor at a permanent disadvantage because of the indivisible nature of the technical package, or whether the poor by-passed the risky trial stage and adapted components tested by others, is hotly debated because of its implications for the relationships between agrarian structure and agricultural growth. The current evidence seems to point in both directions. Later research identified the environmental impacts of increasingly high-energy food-production systems. It has been argued that the emphasis on fertilizer and agrochemicals is misplaced, the former because organic inputs, mulches and slurry are more energy-efficient and can increase food yields at lower cost per unit of energy input, the latter because the application of agrochemicals leads to the pre-emptive evolution of pests, weeds and diseases. Fertilizers have adverse impacts upon the health of human, animal and plant life through nitrification (of nitrates) and eutrophication (of phosphates). In addition, the deployment of pesticides is notorious for poor safety standards. Erosion is taking place in three respects: (1) in the diversity of foods – 75 per cent of plant-derived nutrition is now obtained from eight types of plant; (2) in the gene stock, rendering peasant producers and multinational corporations alike dependent on the gene banks developed through public funding; (3) in soil nutrients and soil structure itself as the environmental sustainability of food production is threatened.

Lipton then turns our attention towards Africa and Latin America and to the second-generation problems besetting staple food research, pointing up the inefficiencies and inequities of starving the very regions and crops which had a low priority in the first round of research funds. Proceeding from evidence for the superior efficiency of small producers and the need for the development of the non-farm economy to be driven by agriculture, Lipton argues for public, non-market funding in order to engender 'market success' in food production. Such research needs to compensate for neglect and for lack of resources rather than reinforce advantage. This means attention to poor people (requiring labour-intensive technology) and their crops (millets, tubers and roots and moisture stress-resistance both in plants and in entire farming systems) in poor regions (the semi-arid and arid tropics, mountains). The 'Hong Kong phenomenon' delinking the attack on poverty from food production is, for Lipton, the exception to prove the rule that, for parts of the world in which agrarian poverty abounds, reliance on specialization and trade would invoke the 'principle of least comparative disadvantage'. Yet developments in biotechnology and associated information technology are not only bypassing such regions (being driven by demand from capital- and energy-intensive monocultural or 'confinement livestock' farming systems), they may (by engineering industrial substitutes for Third World food products) actually reinforce their comparative disadvantage.

The last very prominent production problem concerns the industrialization of food (technically the most dynamic sector in the world), a process which elides agricultural with industrial production and food with feed. The industrial production of food currently absorbs 20 per cent of total energy in industrialized countries and, as Payne says in chapter 5 'is a substantial contributor to . . . global warming'. The relatively stable post-war pattern of production and trade based on protection, on the management of national agricultural surplus production and on the replication of US food policies, is being confounded by the emergence of continentally integrated trading blocs in America, Europe and Asia. Japanese agribusiness has embarked on a distinctive path of global expansion while a new era of corporate freedom (and national debt) has resulted in the appearance of new agricultural countries (NACs). In chapter 10, Friedmann points to an imminent 'second agricultural revolution' in soya and hybrid maize, globally sourced for animal food production, which renders consumption increasingly dependent on an unstable combination of international agribusiness and national and international government regulation. The capacity of nation-states to regulate transnational corporations (TNCs) has, according to Friedmann, been threatened and may be being replaced by competition between states in the provision of incentives to TNCs.

In chapter 9, Buckland tours the frontiers of agribusiness's food research, describing technologies and chemicals for the preservation, fortification and transformation of food, for the replacement of food items by ones having superior nutritional or technical properties, and for new (sometimes inorganic) food sources. The food research frontier is implicitly located in places and at times and in food items where food laws, medical and nutritional science and consumer organizations best support the rapid industrialization of food. At present, for these reasons rather than because of the exigencies of their diet, despite its historical repulsion of the US food industry and because of its national strategy of diversified supplies,[3] the frontiers of food research appear to be in Japan. It is in Japan (where consumers are reacting against the invasion of Western diets they consider 'unhealthy') that the properties of food, drink and medicine are currently being fused in the 'functional drink'. Whether consumers are sovereign, or whether their tastes and values are actively shaped by the food industry in its own interests, is debated by Buckland and Friedmann in chapters 9 and 10, respectively. Yet also worthy of some further comment because of its importance to us as consumers is the development of institutions of food regulation in the industrialization of food production.[4]

States are repositories of guarantees of food safety for their population. In pluralist democracies such as the US and the UK, food regulation has evolved from an origin in the need to control adulteration. Early laws were supported by food manufacturers as a means of eliminating competitors unable to bear the costs of not adulterating. In the UK, modern regulation dates from the 1955 Food and Drugs Act implemented by means of a Food Advisory Committee. Taking additives as an example, regulation requires a 'positive list' of safe chemicals. The way such lists are compiled is of relevance. Food additives have first to be shown to be needed. The 'need' for an additive is not a nutritional matter but refers to the technological need of a food industry. If an additive is deemed to be needed in this way, its safety in use is then ascertained through toxicological evidence scrutinized by a committee of scientific experts and of civil servants from relevant departments. Necessary toxicological research is sponsored by the industrial company interested. The evidence will normally be of one or a combination of three kinds: *in vitro* or animal experiments which present problems of inference to human conditions, and epidemiological research which, by its very nature, is very difficult to conduct. Funds and representatives of food industries are prominent in this regulatory process. By contrast, consumers have no access to information because the regulatory screening is protected under the Official Secrets Act. The regulation of industrial food production in the US differs from that in the UK in that it was formalized earlier and is formally adversarial rather than consensual. Though the Food and Drugs Administration (FDA) referred to by Buckland and Friedmann in chapters 9 and 10 was set up in 1927, it was not until 1960 that the burden of proof of healthy properties was shifted from the FDA to the food industry. Unlike the UK there is greater, though not complete, freedom of information. The FDA has its own resource base for safety testing but the concept of need is not incremental. So many more additives are regulated as safe than in the UK. Nevertheless, under both regulatory systems the positive lists are actually incomplete and, furthermore, the US has a large category of provisionally listed items which may sojourn in this state for decades. Of such bureaucratic regulatory systems it has been said: 'It is not knowledge or skill alone that is wanted of the expert . . . what matters is the halo of impartial prestige his skills give him, allowing him to neutralise conflict laden encounters – between governments, between a government and its governed – and to disguise political issues, for a time, as technical ones',[5] and more extremely: 'Unfortunately the history of every regulatory agency in the US government is that it comes to represent the industry or groups it is supposed to control'.[6] Of growing political influence is thus a view, articulated through consumer movements, that such regulatory systems are 'captured': not only overtly via funding and representation, but more insidiously by infiltration and by the development of regulatory specialists with interests and with a scientific culture common to counterparts in the food industry. We will return to this issue in the last part of this introduction.

Food Distribution

About 11 per cent of grain production crosses international borders. Trade is conventionally modelled as voluntaristic exchange bringing gains to both parties. But it can also be depicted as a type of strategic behaviour under conditions of uncertainty, and then the international food trade is revealed as having a number of awkward characteristics which may prevent mutual gains. First, there are multiple suppliers of food as a raw material who have incomplete information and hazardous agricultural production conditions. As a result suppliers to the world market face relatively unstable and fluctuating prices conducive to error in production and trade decisions. Second, the irreversible process of technical development has generated structural overproduction in certain parts of the world, aided and abetted by a battery of protective devices and considerably high protective ramparts erected for political and social as much as economic reasons.[7] Irritated by the link between debt repayments and international exports, some locked (by the after-effects of Programme Food Aid on the tastebuds of their elites) into importing foodgrains such as wheat in societies producing millet, tubers and rice, Third World suppliers to the international market are not always trading voluntarily. Moreover, they are forced not only to scale the policy fortifications protecting Western economies but also to compete with subsidized exports – 'food-effluents' – from these castellated sites. Third, there is a fallacy of composition in increasing production for international markets of a few commodities defined by comparative advantage, all of which face declining terms of trade as Third World exports tend to do.[8] Forty-two per cent of Third World debt is attributed to adverse terms of trade for the products they export.

There is another story, however, because the dramatis personae of the last paragraph were abstract suppliers (implicitly nation-states) on abstract markets (implicitly competitive ones). In this book, as elsewhere, two stories tend each to be told as though the other did not exist. The actual international food markets, on which what Friedmann calls the 'food regime' operates, can be stylized somewhat differently. These 'markets' tend to be structured not competitively but in oligopolies. One private, export–import house controls 60 per cent of world cereals trade. Almost all primary food commodities are marketed by six trading companies along with over 90 per cent of US exports of wheat, maize and sorghum.

Not only do these firms dominate any given international market, but they have three further characteristics. First, these firms are vertically integrated, structured so as to handle inside the firm a series of trading, shipping and processing activities as well as the agricultural production process itself, increasingly on contract with producers ranging from small peasants to plantations, on terms and conditions fixed with cultivators in advance. Such arrangements bypass 'the market' and reinforce the residual risk-bearing property rights of producers.[9] Over a third of world trade is internalized within transnational corporations. Second, they are horizontally integrated and diversified in their commodity portfolios. Third, they are globally spread in a flexible 'butterfly capitalism'.[10] In Third World market economies food multinationals account on average for 25 per cent of national product and 12 per cent of formal employment. They are the most powerful motor of economic development, to whom the practically immobile national labour markets and resource endowments are enticements, but to whom the nation-state in its role as taxer and regulator appears more often than not as an obstacle. Firms structured in this way, with international hierarchies of shareholders, managers, technical experts, skilled and unskilled labour, are difficult to make accountable even when they can be proved to have transgressed legal boundaries.[11] While international regulation is ostensibly made by states, formidable economic power is actually wielded by these financial, trading and industrial institutions.[12]

One way in which states can and have reacted to multinational capital is by controlling domestic trade themselves. They have also had few alternatives under conditions where lack of infrastructure, and the low densities, small consignments and sporadic periodicities of marketed surplus have repelled trading capital whether it be local or international. This now much criticized state regulation had as its aims and objectives the stabilization of prices paid to producers and charged to consumers, the moulding of production decisions, the engineering of income levels in both the agricultural and non-agricultural sectors, the provision of nutritional safety nets, the guarding of emergency reserves and of more routine buffer stocks to be released seasonally in locations and at times of high prices.

In practice, active intervention has often sown the seeds of its own destruction, with states acting in the private interests of their officials, and with their teratogenic trading organizations growing overcentralized, overmanned, sluggish in decision making, in permanent pitched battle with reserve banks and treasuries over finance and over the subsidies needed to maintain the bureaucratic taste for technological gigantism. In addition, state trading organizations have been frequently burdened with the achievement of social goals as well as profit maximization (or subsidy minimization), with the provision of safety nets for the rural poor which have been transformed into hammocks swung in by privileged urban groups. Governments have also even had difficulty in providing a skeletal regulatory framework involving law and order, property rights and contract enforcement, price information, standardized weights, measures and quality categories without which private markets do not function.

It is not surprising that the policy pendulum swung and that, since the early 1980s, entirely unexamined 'markets' have been invoked as more efficient alternatives. Under conditions where the state has relinquished its previous monopoly, private domestic grain markets have often developed at a disappointing pace and have taken unanticipated forms.[13] And where private domestic markets have been long established, they frequently parade idiosyncracies which economists like to identify as deformations: local monopolies; collusive oligopolies co-existing in a stable relationship with swarms of more or less legal petty trade; trade tied and repeated through narrow and exclusive social networks; social barriers to trade such as gender, religion or caste; commercialization under conditions of coercion; contracts on one market entailing open-ended obligations on one or more others and much else besides.

In the absence of effective state regulation, domestic food merchants in Third World countries have developed their own regulatory bodies. At the same time these institutions (Chambers of Commerce, Grain Associations and so on) are deeply preoccupied with at least two other activities: first, with the reactive lobbying of government at the point of implementation of its interventions, and second, with defensive responses to threats to trading profits by organized labour. They may additionally perform insurance and banking functions for members; or be an avenue for expressions of piety and philanthropy. These regulating institutions are necessary to the development of food markets but they may exclude some traders, they may act at variance with the law and they may exact arbitrary and unjust penalties on those judged miscreants. Food markets of this sort can and do generate high returns to trade and act as arenas for entrepreneurial flair. At the same time they may discriminate against certain kinds of trader and certain kinds of food producer and, in so doing, deprive them of resources with which they might expand their enterprises.

Neither states nor markets can exist without each other. Those countries whose levels of undernutrition are live issues in international politics are precisely those countries where both state and market function with many particularly blatant objectives over and above the logic of economic efficiency.

Consumption and its Pathologies

Whereas the bulk of this introduction has been about production and distribution, the bulk of this book is about consumption. It focuses upon three aspects: (1) the relation of consumption to health and well-being (James, Garrow, and Truswell for the most part considering conditions of abundance in chapters 2, 4 and 3, and Payne tackling conditions of scarcity in chapter 5); (2) its symbolic and political meaning (Mintz, chapter 6) and (3) the role of food consumption in social communication and conflict, evinced here by the ambivalent part played by food in the subordination of women within the household (Whitehead, chapter 7).

A lively concern with beneficial and with harmful properties of food is not a neurotic pathology of affluence but seems a characteristic of all human societies. In affluent societies, and increasingly among the educated elites of poor ones, however, the properties of food which cause or harm health now tend to be established by science. In the West, a statistical or epidemiological approach to the value of food which emphasizes life chances and behaviour has replaced the association of food with morality and, via morality, with immortality. Boyd Orr wrote of nutritional health that its achievement led to a 'state of well being such that no improvement can be effected by a change of diet'.[14] Yet, as James writes in chapter 2, this well-being cannot be defined adequately as a physically measurable freedom from disease; it is experienced as a satisfaction with a state. Scientific ideas are therefore in intimate contact with culture on the many occasions when measurable conditions are translated into a felt experience. Health cannot be ascertained as a benchmark state either for a population or for an individual in terms of genetic potential.

It is as well then to look a little further at an important contribution of post-war food policy and nutritional science to our ideas about essential requirements for nutritional health.[15] It would be useful in a social engineering sense and would no doubt also contribute to our experience of well-being if we could know the quantities of nutrients required for a Boyd Orr state of health. We might also be better judges of the official estimates of those falling short, which currently vary from the World Bank's over one billion to FAO's 477 million. The limitations of scientific evidence on which a full answer needs to be based are well explained by James, Truswell and Garrow in chapters 2, 3 and 4 respectively.

The relationships between human diets and health (unlike those of animals) are both complex and indirect. Their elucidation involves long and indeterminate time lags and much evidence is of the sort which is consistent with more than one interpretation. James, Truswell and Garrow all deconstruct health and consider the history of evidence linking diet with a family of degenerative diseases: coronary heart disease (CHD), cancers, high blood pressure (hypertension) and diabetes. James is at pains to show that protective factors (such as the vitamins and minerals available in fruit and vegetables), thought 50 years ago to prevent trace deficiency diseases, are now thought also to modify the relation between types of saturated fatty acids and cholesterol (and therefore to guard against CHD) and further to maintain the stability and integrity of DNA (and therefore to guard against cancers). Truswell also shows how and why carbohydrate and even sugar have been rehabilitated into therapeutic diets for diabetics and how complex dietary and behavioural responses involving reductions in salt, alcohol and weight are required to reduce hypertension. Garrow provides ample justification for his case that obesity is not only a predisposing, indirect risk factor for these degenerative diseases, but that it also has a direct impact on disease – by reducing sensitivity to insulin, increasing the rate of aging of tissue and, through wear and tear, increasing the risk of musculoskeletal disease. Working backwards from these diseases to crucial nutrients we are shown extremely complex associations, knowledge of the causal mechanisms of which is at present quite rudimentary.

Even if we limit attention to one key nutrient, energy, there are many ambiguities associated with 'essential requirements'. Recommendations (which appear on food labels) are designed to apply to everyone. They are derived either from averages in 'healthy populations' or from a level which covers the consumption of almost everyone (in order to cater for those with over-average needs). These will necessarily also overprovide for almost everyone's 'needs'. Recommendations have not been static. Between 1943 and 1974, the US National Academy of Science reduced calorie requirements by 16 per cent in line with measurements of energy consumption. In India between 1970 and the present, requirements levels have declined by over 20 per cent.[16] For certain nutrients, recommendations are not based on scientific evidence and currently recommended levels owe much to social pressures and values, even to horse trading across expert committees.

In physiological terms, health can be defined as a state of nutritional balance, but there is a range of intakes, metabolic and behavioural responses which might bring about such a balance. If we skirt round notions of equilibrium and instead define physiological health in terms of states of avoidance of undesirable symptoms (such as failure to maintain growth) or unacceptable penalties (such as the involuntary cessation of lactation or unacceptably slow rates of recovery from disease), we are still faced with the problem of specifying desirable and acceptable states and conditions and of applying them to individuals.

Energy is required for three purposes: body maintenance, growth and activity. Energy for body maintenance is the principal component of requirement, even in growing and active children. The standards for the basal metabolic rate (BMR) at which the body ticks over have been obtained from resting American subjects, are conventionally presented for different body weights by sex, and have been found to be set high in relation to BMRs of other populations, for example South Asians. Owing to technical problems in measuring the efficiency of conversion of food into energy, individual requirements are conventionally set at a safe 1.5 BMR or at the lower limit of 1.5×0.8 BMR. Growth standards are set at 5 Kcalories per gramme of tissue gained. Activity is the most varied component of need and the energy requirements of activity vary considerably. Even so, the elusiveness of the requirement here is the result 'merely' of measurement difficulties.

The controversial notion of adaptation challenges the idea of a fixed requirement in a more fundamental way. It is argued that, within thresholds, humans can adapt the efficiency with which they metabolize energy in an entirely benign, autoregulated way; so that people on low energy intakes metabolize it more efficiently and vice versa. The concept of adaptation is further confused by two additional applications: first to behaviour changes (as when a pregnant woman cuts down on heavy work to compensate for the energy needs of her foetus while not increasing her energy intake; or as when weight is deliberately gained in one season so as to lose it in a season of low food supply and heavy work). Second, adaptation may be physiological. The energy-absorbing organs of the body compose different proportions of total body weight as total body weight varies. Thus, the condition of malnutrition elides with that of adaptation and there is considerable indeterminacy in each of our 'essential requirements'. The most obvious corollary is that undernutrition is not easily measured by nutrients intake. As Payne explains in chapter 5, nor can adult smallness *per se* be taken as evidence of current undernutrition, even of the chronic type, for smallness is now understood to be an irreversible genetic response to infectious insults in early childhood. Small stature carries disadvantages for the maximum rate of manual work (which is rarely demanded in the tropics) but otherwise has as yet no known physical disadvantages while it saves calories. Loose definitions of requirements (at one extreme denoting consumption which promotes health and, at the other extreme, consumption which eliminates risk of nutritional disease or death) have tended to lead to untargeted food policy responses by governments. Such interventions conflate less urgent nutritional needs with more urgent ones.

While the nutritional properties of food and the association of food items with health owe much to media obsession in the West, governments also play a crucial promotive role in shaping consumption, principally, in advanced market economies by the light and gentle expedient of education and advice. In Britain, some of the relationships between diet and disease reviewed in chapters 2, 3 and 4 have been processed through government by a series of expert working parties and advisory committees representing a variety of interests (the food industry, public health education, medical and nutritional academics, the Ministry of Agriculture, Fisheries and Food, the Department of Health and Social Security, and so on). As a result, much food is now nutritionally labelled. A stream of goal-oriented, consensual reports have issued forth since 1979 and have merged with professional reports so as to permit official recommendations for changes to dietary patterns. In this process, quantitative goals are known to have suffered modification not because of conflict in science so much as because of conflict in economic interests.

Between 1980 and 1991, British consumption per caput of all food items except cheese, fish, processed fruit and vegetables and (processed) cereals fell. The roles in this transformation played by the media, the government and the food industry are impossible to disentangle, as are their individual effects on 'health'. The case of milk is a good illustration of how public sector health education can act as a midwife to the food industry – in this case to firms producing low fat milk products. Despite increases in purchasing power and a reduction in the real price of milk, demand for milk has declined. In contrast to post-war years when the public was taught that meat and dairy products were good nutritional protectors, that milk was 'good for you', a sizeable minority now believe that milk is 'bad'. Dramatic changes are associated with this change in view though they are by no means solely attributable to it. Soft (and carbonated) drinks have eaten into the slice of the beverage market held by tea, coffee (and milk). From 1980–93 the proportion of all liquid milk which is purchased in semi- or fully skimmed form has soared from negligible to just under half. Health education is part of other social trends. Doorstep deliveries, distinctive to Britain, have been vanquished on the supply side by the 'total provisioning' achieved by supermarkets (and the implication of this – global sourcing – means that supermarket milk products are far from being domestically produced). On the demand side they have been threatened by the incompatibility of doorstep provisioning (and thus doorstep curdling) with women's wage work and by the revolution in convenience foods (where the milk is already added). There are strong class patterns to the response to the regulation of consumption by advice. Healthy diets are least affordable by the poor and the unemployed (even if they know about them) while the prices of the components of healthy diets rise fastest. Women in the social categories of poor and unemployed are known to tend to defer to the dietary preferences of husbands who have 'conservative' and highly patterned food habits.[17] The result of a minimalist approach to the regulation of consumption is the policy paradox that intended beneficiaries become victims.

For the French anthropologist Lévi-Strauss, assuming abundance, 'food is good to eat and good to think with'. The second aspect of consumption – its meaning – is so well explored in this book by Mintz and Whitehead in chapters 6 and 7 respectively, that little needs to be added here. Food has three kinds of meaning. The first sort is symbolic. In examining the idea of requirements above, we have been touching on the dual role of food as cause of harm and as therapy, for in the West science has been invoked to blur the distinction between food and medicine (and now between both of these and drink). What Lin Yutang wrote about Chinese cuisine in 1938 has come to pass far beyond the borders of China:

> Eventually we have to come to a conception of health and disease by which the two merge into each other, when men eat in order to prevent disease instead of taking medicine in order to cure it . . . before that time comes, the distinction between medicine which nourishes the body and medicine which cures disease will have to be abolished.[18]

Yet even in our scientific food cultures, a wide variety of foods 'mean' health. For some it is greens and underpolished rice, while spectators of the 1992 Olympic Games were persuaded by a barrage of television advertising that health resided in the very same brands of chocolate bars, soft carbonated drinks and yoghurts which the first group of healthy consumers would dismiss as 'junk'. And the association with well-being may be elaborate and indirect. In South Asia and elsewhere in the Middle and Far East, foods are experienced first and foremost as hot or cold, a binary classification which has nothing to do with temperature or with hot spice, and seems also to have no consistent biochemical basis. Yet it is this 'heat' which has implications for health and it is this 'heat' which is laden with further qualities – virility, purity, auspiciousness and honour. The symbolic meaning of food far exceeds the medicinal, however medicine is understood. Mintz has shown, for example, how the sweetness of honey and sugar came to connote sweetness of personality.[19] That food is a means of communication does not however mean that food behaves like a verbal language with a grammar and syntax.

The global and historical pervasiveness of a meal pattern made of a starchy core, a flavoursome fringe and a legume communicates a 'common principle' which may still amount in certain societies to a 'governing idiom for life' (the protection of which, in the case of Japan, may have the power to stymie the General Agreement on Tariffs and Trade). So the second meaning of food is social. Society defines food. Whitehead shows in chapter 7 that not all food is Food; that not all eating occasions are Meals and that not all eating may be Eating. Towards the end of his seminal study of the cultural and political history of sugar, Mintz details the ways in which the social connotation of food is changing. He argues in fact that the meal is being desocialized just as food and feeding are being associated with other increasingly varied areas of social life and with an array of simultaneous pleasures. His 'gastroanomie' results from the invasion of eating by institutional provisioning, by global standardization and stylistic internationalization, by food grazing and browsing and by independent eating.[20] At the same time we observe an explosion in the ways in which food is deployed to express identity and seal individuality: even in Anglo-Saxon, middle-class North Oxford, one cannot avoid the epicurean cultures of food; the competitive, anxiety-ridden foodism; the production of ethnic foods with novel technologies and their endowment with novel aesthetics and meaning.

The third meaning is political and concerns the social relations and political arrangements which condition the availability of food. Tobacco, tea and sugar were the first objects within capitalism that conveyed with their use the complex idea that 'one could become different by consuming differently'.[21] And sugar, once the link between slave-based plantation production and the European elite, was transformed over time and with the deepening of industrialization into the working-class necessity it remains to this day. Wheat surpluses, sent not so long ago as food aid for geopolitical reasons ostensibly to the poor of sub-Saharan Africa, are now a necessary commercial import for the elites of those countries. British children's actions of protest aimed against factory farming (aided and abetted by animal rights groups) have had a material impact upon the food purchasing and provisioning patterns of school caterers. Thirty per cent of British schoolchildren are currently vegetarian, though of many subtle persuasions. And so on.

The provision of food, as Whitehead reminds us in chapter 7, is an arena for eloquent statements about status, generosity, honour, purity and power – see her final stories of food and domestic violence, food and retaliation. Nevertheless, the food arena is part of the wider domestic arena wherein families reproduce themselves from generation to generation. Virtually worldwide, women perform in this wider domestic arena according to a paradigm of sexual and culinary service, which is in turn part of the cultural and material system of control known as patriarchy. Payne and Whitehead show that this general sex bias may take on a nutritional expression in South Asia while Lipton observes that such a nutritional disadvantage within the household may be a rational response to gender-based discrimination on markets outside the household (see chapters 5, 7 and 8 respectively). Women then have a comparative advantage in unpaid domestic work and may be fed less well because male wages in the world outside the home are higher than those for women. It is a matter of contested debate, however, whether the comparative advantage of individuals in resource allocation within a household is (1) a cultural matter, a manifestation of patriarchy and not a reflection of a valuation of human beings in crude terms of economic investment; (2) determined materially by gender-neutral markets where the prior duties and obligations of domestic work constrain certain individuals (women, the old) to certain most poorly remunerated tasks; or (3) determined materially by economic markets structured by patriarchy so that women are less well remunerated than men irrespective of their productivity.

Food System Breakdown and Famine

Although the incidence of famine has been on the decline since World War II, famines endure as one of the greatest scandals of the last part of the twentieth century. Until recently they were as taboo on the scientific agenda as death itself is in Western societies. We now know a great deal more about them. Famine is distinguished by mass starvation. It is an extreme phenomenon. As Payne observes in chapter 5, it is different from the undernutrition which is seasonal, chronic and structural. Recent demographic and anthropological research has revealed that our association of famine with food scarcity and elevated mortality rates is usually both inaccurate and ethnocentric. Maximum mortality often occurs some time after the mitigation of food scarcity, when people fall victim to infected water, cholera and when malaria reappears. Famine is understood by those who endure it not as signifying death through starvation so much as extreme scarcity of vital elements of social life: not only food, but sex, status, honour.[22] Death is a distant and sometimes patterned event during famine, more likely for some classes than others, and for some age and gender groups than others. It is a vivid signpost to a social breakdown caused by failure of the system of production, distribution and consumption.

That famines resulted from failures of food production seemed so obvious that it has taken years to be thoroughly questioned. It is still the assumption upon which the FAO monitors national food availability and triggers international relief. 'There being not enough food'[23] is likely still to figure as a cause of famines in isolated regions of subsistence production dependent upon fickle rainfall. Such conditions are rare now. Payne explains in chapter 5 that in the long sweep of history, however, physiological and behavioural responses have provided a 'feedback' link whereby the current density of a population influences the subsequent reproductive performance of individual members, 'resulting in populations' regulating themselves at levels below the maximum that the ecological niche supplying food could sustain without irreparable damage'. Even then, famine has not been a purely natural disaster but has resulted from the failure of social coping mechanisms. Population pressures on fragile environments, the failure to conserve moisture, increased demand for water, the privatization and commercialization of common property resources, and state taxation systems which lead to overgrazing, are all examples of social activity which increases the vulnerability of food production to maldistribution of rainfall or to drought and, *mutatis mutandis*, to flood.

But we have already relaxed the Crusoe assumptions. Our understanding of famine has been massively enhanced by the jolt given to the subject by Amartya Sen's distinction between a failure of supply and a failure of demand or, as he develops it, of entitlement.[24] Famine happens according to Sen because of people's not having enough food. Their entitlement to food can result from what they own or from what they can command from exchange on markets. Starvation results from critically adverse changes in the terms of exchange of specific social groups, when the capacity to produce what is exchanged for food atrophies or when prices of goods sold by non-food producers slump – their own labour, their cloth, their draught animals. Sen musters persuasive cases to show that production need not fail nor staple food prices rise for there to be famine.

But this is also not the whole story. One of the great strengths of Sen's theory is that his markets are competitive and efficient. But famines can also be caused by market failures in conditions where money demand for food exists but food does not reach it. The kind of strangely structured and poorly behaved markets described earlier and common in underdeveloped agrarian economies may fail to deliver food because of lack of systems of communication and transport, or because traders perceive the response (either by themselves or by them in concert with others yet unknown) as excessively risky in relation to the likely returns, or markets may fail as a result of hoarding in an over-reaction to incorrect information about food scarcity.

The notion of entitlement resonates with legal overtones which direct us to a non-market source of entitlement – the state, whose legitimacy, as we have seen, is often judged (not only by outsiders but also domestically) by its guarantee of food and water. Failure to compensate for food market failure may cause famines. This kind of state failure will result from the breakdown of rules of access which, more often than not, take different forms in practice from those specified in formal bureaucratic procedure. But the state may fail in two further sectors and thereby create famine. New research questioning the predictions of entitlement theory has emphasized a public health explanation for famine. In Sudan in the 1980s, the state failed to provide potable water. Entitlement failures did not cause death but recourse to inadequate and contaminated water supplies did, and it muddied the social profile of the victims.[25] Lastly, war-famines may be seen as spectacular examples of state and market failures. War disrupts food production, supplies, distribution and relief. It deflects resources from economic development and welfare provision and it displaces consumers.

The other non-market social arenas whose failure may cause famine are the household and the various redistributivist institutions of local society (livelihood guarantees, harvest sharing, relations of patronage, and so on).

The word enfranchisement has been invoked for these circumstances of customary non-market claim.[26] Relations of enfranchisement within household or locality then also define peoples' access to both markets and state. When 'custom' diverges from 'law', people tend to engage in struggle for their customary practice.[27] It is being realized that, under conditions of food stress, such customary practices or enfranchisements collapse. Under famine conditions, peoples' survival strategies are sequenced. Assets which perform the function of savings and insurance are marketed for food first, while assets which generate income are relinquished last. In South Asian societies, the former tend to be owned by women while the latter are owned by men. Relationships of patronage are replaced by contracts which exclude non-market obligations on the part of employers. The collapse of individual enfranchisement within the household has been argued to result when the household patriarch can no longer sustain the patriline; or, by way of contrast, when local entitlements or enfranchisements fail to provide subordinate and dependent family members with viable subsistence – reasons for them to co-operate within the household – at which point they are shed. The two lines of argument have opposite implications for famine relief, the first leading to livelihood provision for males, the second for females.[28]

In sum, though it may be inconvenient to sacrifice an attachment to one explanation, it is more useful to assume that modern famines are concatenation processes than otherwise. As Payne writes, the genesis of famine is varied and so also will be its impact. Famine is also an attenuated process rather than an event, one in which there are beneficiaries as well as losers. That famine policy currently concentrates on the final stage, on victims and on relief, is an eloquent testimony to poverty of resolve. It is to this question of resolve that we now turn.

What is to be Done?

Robert Kates, the Director of the Brown University 'World Hunger Program', has recently made a statement which is painful in its honesty about advocacy, concluding: 'Not only is it difficult to pursue a credible science, but it is even more difficult to be an effective social policy advocate'.[29] In attempting to sort out the reasons for such a situation, he reveals the intellectual corruption that academic research strains to avoid in its dialogue with social policy and politics. Anyone who has had reason to query social welfare law in Britain or elsewhere knows that the state, perforce, is a road-roller rather than a high performance sports car. In Kates' case, the translation of research to policy confronts the fact, also emphasized in this introduction and in this book, that research produces arrays of answers to questions, arrays of solutions to problems. Further, for research to enter the policy arena, presentational procedure is paramount. Kates identified as crucial in the advocacy work of his particular programme the choices between advocacy of incremental or fundamental directed change, optimistic or pessimistic advocacy. Selective and contingent use of evidence is unavoidable. Low estimates of the malnourished make the problem appear tractable, high estimates may produce a counsel of despair. It is evident that what he calls the 'hunger industry' is not simply a political technocracy in its own right; it has its own internal politics.

Running the risk of an arbitrary oversimplification, and mindful of the facts (1) that the social policy advocacy of individual academics may not fit neatly into the classification below, and (2) that there is at the time of writing no viable alternative to market economy, the hunger industry's political battle lines appear currently to be as follows:

(1) The World Bank and International Monetary Fund's conditions on their major stabilization and structural adjustment loans require the national liberalization and deregulation of production and marketing of food and the compression of the territory of active government intervention to a minimum. The protracted Uruguay Round of the General Agreement on Tariffs and Trade (GATT) aims to achieve similar goals internationally and globally, based on reasoning about comparative advantage, gains to trade, efficiency losses from subsidies and both efficiency and equity losses from protection. Such arguments, supported by elaborate counterfactual modelling,[30] fail to address the contradiction between ostensibly democratic international decision making and the opposition to such liberalization based, quite logically, on the very same reasoning and modelling by numerous countries such as the Third World food-importing epicentres of poverty and malnutrition, all consistently predicted to be net welfare losers from liberalization. Such arguments also involve assumptions about the efficiency of domestic and international markets which, as we have seen here, are of limited practical usefulness.

(2) At the same time, the World Bank argues for and disburses modest loans for the so-called 'human face' of structural adjustment – a 'New Poverty Agenda'. This consists of safety nets, which are increasingly highly specified in the military metaphor of targeting – health, educational, nutritional and social security safety nets – involving technology-driven, livelihood-generating, diversified development which is targeted towards disadvantaged regions. The New Poverty Agenda is based on reasoning about the equity and 'human capital efficiency' gains of successful targeting, which is in turn based on somewhat heroic assumptions about the will and the capacity of government (1) to target at all and (2) to target cost-effectively.[31]

(3) A view, from many scholars of Development Studies (and influential in the United Nations Development Programme and the UN's World Institute for Development Economics Research), that privatization and 'marketization' is neither always necessary nor sufficient to 'beat persistent hunger and deprivation', since markets respond to wants rather than needs. Such developmental goals are most rapidly achieved not so much by growth-mediated welfare as by immediate and direct investment in social welfare, public health and income support under conditions where public action means not only action by governments, but also ownership and participation by the public (with special attention to female members of the public).[32] Such conclusions draw on historical evidence from advanced and underdeveloped countries and from a variety of political systems and regimes, even though the optimal environment is clearly a pluralist political system which combines collaboration and adversarial politics (for which there are few historical examples).

(4) A broad church of advocacy supported by the United Nations Research Institute for Social Development and by many researchers in non-governmental organizations (NGOs), arguing not only for the desirability of undogmatic and flexible responses to 'hunger' but also stressing the importance of reforms to the structures of ownership of assets and land, respect for 'peoples' knowledge', sustainability in food production, environmental protection, the development of participative social movements and of new forms of popular accountability (peasant associations, political parties, trades unions, co-operatives, women's groups, secularist groups, consumer movements, public health and environmental groups and legal awareness groups, and so on), the decentralization of trade, reforms in the functioning and accountability of developmental institutions of the United Nations and the need to improve national and global regulation of the industrial production of food.[33] The latter may involve protectionist policies which puts this school most squarely at loggerheads with the first in our list. This form of advocacy is based on assumptions that economies and societies are best understood in terms of both inequalities of interests and conflicts of interest and that the raising of welfare implied by the optimistic metaphor of 'development' involves confronting and changing the very power relations with which this broad school is either not usually in immediate contact, or is often prevented by charity laws from challenging.

The expert contributors to this volume have suggested a variety of ways in which problems with food might be addressed. Mindful of the need for caution about the social role of experts in masking political problems as technical ones (a process helped in the English language as nowhere else by a verbal distinction between policy and politics which enables advocacy to be depoliticized), the main thrusts are as follows.

In chapter 2, James argues from evidence on adult under- and malnutrition that nutritional priorities need to be reorganized so that the current bias towards child and maternal nutrition be rectified by attention to all adults, with the emphasis on South Asia rather than Africa and with micro- as well as macronutritional therapies given prominence. For this set of long-term priorities, research on sustainable food production technologies is crucial. All schools of advocacy save the third will have recommendations for different means to achieve this latter objective. In chapter 8, Lipton develops its implications by pointing to the currently stingy funding for agricultural research for research-poor agro-ecological environments, for poor peoples' crops, crop mixes and crop-livestock mixes and by justifying real increases in research resources. Payne has taken a similar view on nutritionally relevant agricultural research in chapter 5. These are convincingly justified inputs into the second school's New Poverty Agenda. In chapter 10, Friedmann takes on the reasoning behind the first battle line in the 'hunger industry' (juxtaposing this with her interest-based reasoning of the stakes involved in international food politics and of the role of multinational corporations which is ignored by the first battle line) and counterargues that international liberalization under GATT may increase the instability of production and trade. Hence her prescription, which protagonists of the first strategy will find unreasonable, for regional autarky and for a community-based politics of food regulation. Such presently utopian, strategic, political argument will have to be scrutinized in any quest to supply responses to Payne's demand for research on the health implications of a globally sustainable diet under conditions of an 'acceptable degree of equity'.

Truswell and Garrow pay attention to issues of resource distribution within affluent societies in chapters 3 and 4, pointing to the need to address the class profiles both of obesity – the key predisposing factor to diseases of diet under conditions of affluence – and of the social compulsion to diet. With respect to underdeveloped societies, Payne dissociates himself from the view that nutrition programmes can act as social and economic catalysts and thereby disguise the political process as a technical one. Limited nutritional ('technical') gains from existing food distribution programmes require comprehensive and overt supplementation by increased access (or improved entitlement) not only to food, but to free, feminized and decentralized health services and to primary and basic education. This is strong endorsement for the third battle line. While endorsing the feasibility of targeted policy on the whole which can be implemented in the absence of the structural change advocated by the fourth school, Payne also draws attention to the distinction between highly targeted policies (based on precise nutritional aetiology) which address chronic (if seasonal) levels of nutritional deprivation below which victims run the risk of death, and other much broader social policies of the third school type (which are less precise about cause and circumstance and which have the effect of establishing decent standards of food consumption). As an example of the latter type of policy, he uses the costs of micronutrient fortification (advocated by James in chapter 2), particularly the hidden systemic costs of effective delivery.

It is ironic that the supply of advocacy in this book is by food consumers and vicariously on behalf of other food consumers, whereas the institutional demand for advocacy is from development banks and from governments which have historically been preoccupied not with consumption but with production, upon whose performance both financial loans and their repayment depend. In the interstices is a less examined area of policy which this chapter has tried to introduce. This is the regulation of the corporate capital which controls global distribution. On this subject, consider the following statement echoing the thrust of Buckland's argument in chapter 9:

> Biotechnology can be a major contributor . . . [to feeding] all those hungry mouths . . . providing that society, governments and industry can work together . . . We're in the food business to make money. A lot of the third world can't afford to buy our first wave of products. We hope that in the second wave our products, ideas and technology can be transferred either directly to the third world or through those breeding institutions that support them.[34]

The screening of such ideas, technology and products is the responsibility of national, and international regulatory bodies. In theory, regulation is achieved by three means: first, simply by increasing competition; second, by fiat (by rules about matters such as price, safety in the workplace, quality standards, the characteristics of products, pollution and other externalities) imposed on monopolies awaiting the arrival of competitors; and third, by fiat imposed regardless of the type of competitive environment. Not least because of a lack of theoretical consensus about optimal institutional ways to regulate corporate capital, it is common that this process tends to be unsystematic, itself in turn unpoliced and vulnerable to the interplay of different and competing interests. We have moved on here to consider not just what is to be done, but how it might be done and the final objective of this introduction is briefly to comment on means and justifications.

How and Why?

How it is done? As a matter of routine, external agents such as banks and United Nations Agencies (not to mention multinational corporations) impose on countries conditions which clearly infringe their sovereignty and their right to self-determination. In so doing, they expose the fragility of an international morality based on equal rights and on the power of nation-states. Behind 'the ebb and flow of current politics and economic struggles lie legal and institutional structures'[35] with ethical bases which may not be very secure. Our enquiry into food finishes, therefore, with two analytical and normative discussions of law and ethics in relation to food.

One of the areas of international law which has been recognized as 'fundamental' is the welfare right to be free from hunger. This right has to be translated from the pious (or cynical) signatures of at least 74 states into operational procedure prior to any institutionalization enabling the adjudication of breaches of law. With regard to the rights to food and to be free from hunger, the first stage of operationalization has only been established, ironically, for conditions of war. This quite shocking absence of progress is not due to the manifest absence of consensus on whether any rights do or need exist, for the widespread signing of two international covenants suggests that welfare rights are conceded. As Alston sees it in chapter 11, the problem of implementation starts with the massive scope of the relevant articles of the covenant on economic, social and cultural rights. (These include the use of science to improve the production, distribution and consumption of food, and the administration of agrarian reform, all in such a way and to such an extent as to realize rights to food.) The problem of implementation then proceeds through the vagueness of specification of beneficiaries or claimants, either as individuals or as nation-states. The convention also ducks the issue of the status of the liberty rights of states to be free from interference from others. Alston's vivid and tragic illustration of the law as an unruly arena of social interpretation builds a case for a start to be made with a legal convention specifying the 'normative implications of the right to food', on which the rest of the process of workability rests.

O'Neill's response in chapter 12 is that, before such a very particular convention is possible, it is necessary to develop an ethical theory of obligation from which an obligation towards those deprived of food can be derived. Her chapter destroys any illusions about the ease of such a project. She argues finally that an obligation to act requires there to be general principles of obligation, and, for these to be possible, there has to be a prior commitment to develop what Sen has called 'capabilities to function'[36] in all members of society. In the absence of such capacities, the principles of obligation cannot be developed. This argument forms the basis of a requirement for redistributive action: 'to refrain from making a principle . . . denying . . . the help needed for agency to survive'.[37] It is a moot point, however, whether her further argument, that those deprived of food are also (except in the very rare case of very extreme deprivation)[38] deprived of the capacity to act as rational, social and moral agents, is historically sustainable.

That moral philosophy cannot give an indisputably correct account of justice, and further that 'obligation and respect cannot be compelled like military power',[39] does not render these concepts redundant. Nor does it prevent action in the direction of improving what are, admittedly, imperfect obligations, both at the formal level of governments and at an individual level within the social and spatial territories in which we each exercise responsibility. Such actions can take a multiplicity of forms – our own compromises within the spheres of the affective and political.

NOTES

1 Cited in Mintz, S. (1985) *Sweetness and Power*, New York, Viking Penguin, p. 4.
2 Pinstrup-Andersen, P. and Hazell, P. (1985) 'The impact of the Green Revolution and prospects for the future', *Food Reviews International* 1(1), 1–25.
3 Japan's strategy of minimal investment and diversified sourcing leads to foreign competition for her import markets (see chapter 10 in this volume).
4 Our discussion of regulation owes much to Abraham, J. (1991) *Food and Development: the political economy of hunger and the modern diet*, London, World Wildlife Fund/Kogan Page.
5 Adams, A. (1979) 'An open letter to young researcher', *African Affairs* 78, 451–79.
6 Judge Lee Loevinger, Head of the US Justice Department's Antitrust Division, in Harris, R. (1964) *The Real Voice*, New York, Macmillan, p. 154; see also the *Guardian*, 12 May 1993, on financial links between the UK Food Advisory Committee and food companies.
7 Protection takes forms of tariffs, quotas, sanitary and phytosanitary precautions and environmental standards. These are unevenly implemented. The proportion of revenue to the food staples producer which came from protection in the early 1980s averaged 42 per cent for the EEC, 16 per cent for the USA and 59 per cent for Japan (OECD National Policies and Agricultural Trade – Country Reports, in Peters, G. H. (1988) 'The interpretation and use of producer subsidy equivalents', *Oxford Agrarian Studies* 17, pp. 186–213).
8 The terms of trade comprise the secular relationship between agricultural and industrial prices – in this case on the world markets. For details, see Fortin, C. (1988) 'International commodities and Third World development: trends and prospects', in O. Stokke (ed.) *Trade and Development: experiences and challenges*, Osle, EADI (European Association of Development Institutes) Book Series, no. 7.
9 Transnational corporations rather rarely enter into contracts with co-operatives, collectives or state farms.
10 Watts, M. (1990) 'Peasants under contract: agro food complexes in the Third World', in H. Bernstein, B. Crow, M. Mackintosh and C. Martin (eds) *The Food Question*, London, Earthscan, pp. 149–62. Watts details examples of abrupt termination or cancellation of contract, of flight of TNCs and of their occasional replacement by state trading institutions in Central America and sub-Saharan Africa.
11 Bartlett, R. (1989) *Power and Economics*, Cambridge, Cambridge University Press.
12 See Buttel, F. (1990) 'Biotechnology and agricultural development in the Third World', in Bernstein et al. (eds) *The Food Question*, pp. 163–80; Benz, H. (1990)

Le riz américain face au marché mondial, Lyons, RONGEAD (Réseau des Organisations Non-Gouvernementales Européenes d'Aide et Développement), for rice; and Gilmore, R. (1982) *A Poor Harvest: the clash of policies and interests in the grain trade*, New York and London, Longman, for wheat.

13 Harriss, B. and Crow, B. (1992) 'Twentieth-century free trade reform', in M. Wuyts, M. Mackintosh and T. Hewitt (eds) *Development Policy and Public Action*, Oxford, Oxford University Press, pp. 199–230.

14 In Pacey, A. and Payne, P. R. (1985) (eds) *Agricultural Development and Nutrition*, London, Hutchinson, p. 46.

15 Our discussion draws on that in Pacey and Payne (eds) *Agricultural Development and Nutrition*, pp. 37–72.

16 Cutler, P. (1984) 'The measurement of poverty: a review of attempts to quantify the poor with special reference to India', *World Development* 12 (11–12), 1119–30; Pacey and Payne (eds) *Agricultural Development and Nutrition*, p. 84.

17 Wheeler, E. (1985) 'To feed or to educate: labelling in targeted nutrition interventions', in G. Wood (ed.) *Labelling in Development Policy*, London, Sage, pp. 133–42; and Houliston, S. (1992) 'The liquid milk market in the UK', M.Sc. Dissertation, Oxford, International Development Centre. Buckland shows in chapter 9 of this volume how low fat spreads follow similar consumption trends to those of skimmed milk.

18 Lin Yutang (1938) *The Importance of Living*, London, Heinemann, pp. 270–1.

19 See Mintz, *Sweetness and Power*. As with health, so the concept of satisfaction or satiety is also object of a range of definitions – even in this volume. For Garrow (ch. 4), satiety is conditioned behaviour. Judgement of satiety is therefore threatened by novelty and by variety which are, as Garrow argues, the prime causes of obesity. For Mintz (ch. 6), satiety comes from palatability, and, for Buckland (ch. 9), it is derived from texture ('mouthfeel'); the health consequences of satiety are, Mintz argues, unknown and, according to Buckland, unproblematical.

20 Mintz, *Sweetness and Power*; see also ch. 6.

21 Mintz, *Sweetness and Power*, p. 185.

22 De Waal, A. (1990) *Famine that Kills*, Oxford, Oxford University Press; Dyson, T. (1991) 'On the demography of South Asian famines', *Population Studies* 45, 1–25 and 279–97.

23 Sen, A. (1980) 'Famines', *World Development* 8 (9), 614.

24 Sen, A. K. (1981) *Poverty and Famines*, Oxford, Clarendon Press; further developed in Drèze, J. and Sen, A. K. (1989) *Hunger and Public Action*, London, Oxford University Press.

25 De Waal, *Famine that Kills*.

26 Appadurai, A. (1984) 'How moral is South Asia's economy? – A review article', *Journal of Asian Studies* XLIII(3), 481–97.

27 Gore, C. (1993) 'Entitlement relations and unruly social practices: a comment on the work of Amartya Sen', *Journal of Development Studies* 29(3), 429–60.

28 Greenough, P. (1982) *Prosperity and Misery in Modern Bengal: the famine of* 1943–1944, London, Oxford University Press; Agarwal, B. (1990) 'Social security and the family', in S. E. Ahmed, A. K. Sen, J. Drèze and N. Stern (eds) *Social Security in Developing Countries*, London, Oxford University Press, pp. 171–245.

29 'Divisions in the Hunger Industry', *Times Higher Educational Supplement*, 16 April 1993, p. 16.
30 Tyres, R. and Anderson, K. (1988) 'Liberalising OECD agricultural policies in the Uruguay Round', *Journal of Agricultural Economics* 39, 2.
31 World Bank (1992) *Poverty Handbook*, Washington, DC, World Bank.
32 Drèze and Sen, *Hunger and Public Action*; see also Cornia, A., Jolly, R. and Stewart, F. (1988) *Structural Adjustment with a Human Face*, London, Oxford University Press.
33 Articulated in Barraclough, S. (1991) *An End to Hunger*, London, Zed Press. Barraclough also puts a well-argued case for subjecting these grand strategies to a rigorous comparison of the dilemmas that they entail when applied to given practical circumstances. See also Lang, T. (1993) *Protecting the Future: the case for the new protectionism and against free trade*, London, Earthscan.
34 Dr Edward Dart, Research Director of ICI Seeds, quoted in Abraham, *Food and Development*, ch. 4, p. 160.
35 O'Neill, O., chapter 12 in this volume.
36 Sen, A. K. (1985) *Commodities and Capabilities*, Amsterdam, North-Holland.
37 O'Neill, O., chapter 12 in this volume.
38 Though there is no reason not to use this argument.
39 Toye, J. (1988) *Dilemmas of Development*, Cambridge, Cambridge University Press, p. 142.

FURTHER READING

Drèze, J. and Sen, A. K. (1991) (eds) *The Political Economy of Hunger*, 3 vols, London, Oxford University Press.

Hazell, P. and Ramasamy, C. S. (1991) (with others) *Green Revolution Revisited*, Baltimore, Johns Hopkins University Press.

Lipton, M., with Longhurst, R. (1989) *New Seeds and Poor People*, London, Unwin Hyman.

Tansey, G. and Worseley, A. (1994) *From Farm to Mouth: a rough guide to the food system*, London, Oxford University Press.

Watts, M. (1983) *Silent Violence*, Berkeley, London, University of California Press.

World Bank (1991) *World Development Report: Poverty*, Washington, DC, World Bank.

2

The Nature of Food: Essential Requirements

Philip James

Nutritional issues are re-emerging as fascinating problems in the biological sciences and involve the most modern aspects of biochemistry and molecular biology. This renewed interest has also been stimulated by the sudden prominence given to nutrition by the British government as it seeks to combat the high rates of a range of chronic diseases in adults. The dietary basis for these diseases is now a tenet of policy making and new proposals suggest that it is the population's behaviour, particularly in relation to diet, which contributes substantially to premature death. Yet few senior doctors and scientists of distinction seem to accept these views; this may be an interesting reflection not only of their education but also of the assumptions of post-war food policies which have pervaded governmental, economic, social and academic thinking for 50 years. To understand this unusual turn of events, it is important to recognize how recently we have acquired the elementary principles of nutrition which led, during World War II, to our current concepts of a 'balanced' diet.

In the early part of this century there was a growing recognition that we needed to avoid deficiency diseases by consuming a variety of foods; a paucity of an individual mineral or vitamin in one food would be balanced by an abundance of the specific micronutrient in another food. The concept of balance was based, therefore, on avoiding deficiency diseases and the population was educated to understand the importance of 'protective foods'. One of the best ways of achieving this seemed to require eating substantial amounts of meat and dairy products so that all the deficiencies, including energy and protein lack, could be prevented. The application of these concepts of variety and balance were later misapplied, so that our current 'balanced' diet, which does indeed avoid all recognized nutritional deficiencies, is now linked to Britain's having the highest rate of premature deaths in the Western world.

The First Revolution in Nutritional Science

We have seen three nutritional revolutions this century, the first relating to the discovery of the essential micronutrients and the avoidance of deficiency diseases. The second was the post-war revolution in nutritional research which then concentrated on animal and food production. The third is newly emerging and recognizes the role of diet in the development of a number of chronic diseases in adult life. By understanding the sequence of thinking in national priorities, we can readily see why we are now in a fascinating phase of transition.

The concept that diseases could be of dietary origin goes back to the Greeks, but the specificity of citrus to cure scurvy was one of the earliest controlled trials carried out by Captain Lind on his long sea voyages. Sailors given limes rapidly recovered from scurvy. This simple remedy had to wait until 1720, however, for Kramer in Austria to introduce it for routine use in the army. Takaki, the Japanese general, linked beri-beri in his troops to their exclusive consumption of polished rice and Eijkman demonstrated the protective role of cereal bran in combating a similar syndrome in chickens. The concept of amines vital to health had led Funk to suggest that there were biologically active 'vitamines' in minute amounts in the diet. Gowland Hopkins, Professor of Biochemistry at Cambridge, undertook a series of carefully controlled studies which confirmed that vital factors of a non-amine form were crucial to the health and growth of animals. Eijkman and Hopkins were awarded Nobel Prizes for their descriptions of the compounds now designated as vitamins. Thus, at the time when biochemistry was an emerging science, nutrition was a principal focus of academic interest. Nutritional interests gained respectability when Mellanby, famous for his research on the effects of diet and fat-soluble factors in the development of bone disease and rickets in pups, was appointed the first Secretary of the Medical Research Council. McCarrison in India linked dietary studies in animals and man by comparing the effects of feeding Sikh and British diets to rats. Rats on British diets failed to grow as well as those on Sikh diets rich in vegetables and fruit.

In Britain, great public concern had arisen during and after the Boer War because so many candidates for recruitment to the army, particularly from the north of England and Scotland, were short, thin and seemed too unhealthy and puny to provide the right quality of fighting man which Britain needed to control its Empire. Since many of these rejected young men came from large working-class families, it was feared that the genetic stock of the British would deteriorate as the numbers of working-class people multiplied more rapidly than the tall, healthy and self-evidently intelligent upper and aristocratic classes! However, the first Director of the Rowett Institute, Boyd Orr, conducted analogous studies to those of Corry Mann[1] where groups of children of different heights were supplemented with single food items to see whether they would show a growth response similar to that seen in animals. Corry Mann's data revealed that short children supplemented with milk grew in height and weight whereas butter and sugar supplements were useful aids to weight rather than height gain. Petty has recalculated Corry Mann's data to reveal that the shortest children responded best.[2] Boyd Orr, with his son-in-law David Lubbock, conducted a survey of the health, dietary practice and purchasing power of working-class households sampled from many different areas of Britain. This led to the publication of *Food, Health and Income* in 1936,[3] which set out the link between poverty, a poor diet, children's short stature and their parents' poor physique and health.

Boyd Orr then campaigned for a change of national strategy and promoted milk as an important item in the diet which should be given to pregnant and nursing mothers and to their children. School milk and school lunches were also proposed as appropriate national schemes for which government had responsibility. Voluntary groups promoted milk drinking and these campaigns were backed by the newly organized Milk Marketing Boards which were desperately seeking an outlet for their dairy farmers' excess produce. This happy conjunction of consumer needs, national health priorities and the requirements for agricultural development had, however, only a modest impact on a government anxious to limit its public spending. Only in 1940 did the potential collapse of war-time food supplies precipitate a remarkably intense, varied and sustained governmental drive to develop coherent national policies which linked agricultural production to health issues.

All may still have come unstuck if the initial policies on food rationing proposed by Whitehall had been accepted. They sought to develop a scheme which would allow specific items of diet to be purchased. Thus, the more affluent sector of the community would have been able to afford a varied diet rich in meat, milk and butter. However, Boyd Orr and Lubbock (personal communication), with their Carnegie Survey on diet and health, were able to convince officials and, presumably, Lord Wooton that equity in availability was vital to the welfare of the working class on whom Britain's war-time success depended. There emerged a rationing system and social policy which became the envy of the world. The British Ministries of Food and Health thereby earned the extraordinary distinction of the Lasker Award, given by the American Public Health Association after the war for their contributions to public health![4]

The Second Revolution

When Boyd Orr left the Rowett Institute to establish the United Nation's Food and Agriculture Organization (FAO), the world was clear about what the priorities were – to produce far more meat, milk and other dairy products, such as butter, so that diets would have enough energy, protein, minerals such as calcium, and vitamins to prevent any deficiency diseases. Children needed these foods to grow well and diets were to provide adults with sufficient energy for the varied physical demands of their work and for their active lives at home. The spectacular successes of war-time policies, the improved growth of children, and reduced morbidity of the population all confirmed that the fundamental principles of human dietary needs had now been established. The problem was how to grow enough food. Millions of refugees in Europe and the Middle East emphasized the fundamental importance of food supplies which, for Britain, had been particularly acute at the outbreak of war since it depended on cheap food imported from the colonies for 70 per cent of its needs. The German submarines had failed to starve Britain into submission, but the nation had been helped by the surge in home-grown food which increased from 30 per cent to 60 per cent or more of total food needs by 1944. Everybody, from royalty downwards, had been mobilized to improve agricultural production. The dairy industry was now struggling to cope, not with the excess milk supplies but with the huge demand for milk, most of which had to be assigned to special feeding programmes for children and mothers.

With the advent of the Cold War, the submarine threat was renewed and the priorities were clear – to increase food production, particularly of animal products, and to produce food as cheaply as possible. This would allow the working class access to a varied and nutritious diet at a price they could afford.

Then began the agricultural revolution with perhaps the most effective collaboration between scientists, industry and policy makers ever achieved in Britain or elsewhere. The Rowett Institute again rapidly expanded with the dissuasion of its second medically qualified Director, David Cuthbertson, from furthering his renowned research on the metabolic response to infection and trauma. His responsibility was to convert the Rowett into an exclusively agricultural institute geared to improvements in animal husbandry. His successor, the late Kenneth Blaxter, became the first non-medical animal nutritionist to be appointed Director and, with his guidance and drive, improvements in animal feeding were progressive and substantial. The priority for agricultural research to allow increased agricultural production was so great, however, that many more institutes were established to cope with demand. By the time I assumed the directorship in 1982, the Rowett was one of 34 agricultural institutes in Britain, 14 of which were developing and assessing new ideas in animal feeding. The cost of meat, milk and butter fell progressively as the Ministries of Agriculture subsidized capital farm improvements, paid for the research and development costs of agriculture and supported a sophisticated network of extension officers to improve the earning power and efficiency of the farming community.

Post-war Britain had seen a collapse of research in human nutrition. The Medical Research Council (MRC) did fund their Ugandan and Jamaican units to contribute to knowledge of the colonies' nutritional needs and how best to combat the prevalence of childhood malnutrition. But in Britain, outstanding scientists such as Hans Krebs, who had contributed so much to war-time research on vitamin and mineral requirements, moved back to their more exciting fields of general biochemistry. McCance's unit in Cambridge was run down, Platt's unit at Mill Hill was closed, and only the Dunn Nutrition Laboratory remained to carry out esoteric research on such problems as the nature of vitamin D metabolism.

The Third Revolution: Diet-related Diseases of Affluent Societies

Although it was only in 1991 that the British government recognized in any integrative way that many of the chronic diseases of adults have a major dietary basis, in practice 100 government reports from different countries have been published which, without exception, emphasize the role of diet in the development of obesity, high blood pressure, coronary heart disease (CHD) and some forms of cancer.[5] The conclusions are surprisingly consistent, given the complex array of evidence from animal, *in vitro*, clinical and epidemiological studies. It is now accepted that diet does affect individuals' metabolism and the pathophysiological processes which lead to several common diseases. Individuals are indeed different by virtue of their genetic inheritance and behavioural idiosyncracies, but the pervading feature of the development of these diseases is the interaction of the genome with the inflow of dietary components whose actions we now recognize as both subtle and varied. Given the interplay of many factors in processes which operate for decades before the clinical picture of heart disease or cancer emerges, it is not surprising that scientists, used to isolating single factors to study in the laboratory, find the role of diet difficult to accept. The concepts are so different from the pre-war issues of simple and specific deficiency diseases where a clear clinical picture develops and then responds rapidly to the provision of the deficient vitamin or mineral. The concepts of prevention are seen to relate to the inexact 'soft' sciences which seem so uncertain compared with the clear diagnostic and therapeutic approaches which dominate much of modern medical practice.

A real problem is how to develop a public health approach where there is considerable uncertainty about the disease mechanisms but sufficient evidence to warrant social changes and legislation to promote preventive measures. The best example of this was the development of the anti-smoking campaigns with legislation on tobacco advertising based on the recognition that smokers developed a range of diseases, including lung cancer, by unknown mechanisms. Complex analyses attempted to identify the relative risks of cigarette, cigar and pipe smoking and long-term studies were needed to assess the benefits of giving up smoking. Nevertheless, most scientists were willing to accept the arguments because there seemed to be a clear link between smoking and disease; the effect was graded in relation to the amount smoked; the relationship was deemed consistent in many studies throughout the world; and, at least for lung cancer, the links were biologically plausible because cigarette tar contained compounds which experimentally could induce marked cellular changes and produce cancer when painted on the skin of susceptible animals. In practice, studies on the relationship between smoking and both heart disease and hypertension were not consistent in all parts of the world (discussed later in this chapter) and only recently have much more complex analyses shown how remarkably damaging smoking really is.[6] Nevertheless, the concept was sufficiently plausible for governments to take action, despite an intensive rearguard of criticism, data manipulation and lobbying by the tobacco industry.[7] It is much more difficult to assign blame to dietary factors than it is to smoking because the first nutritional revolution conditioned everyone to believe that foods were beneficial and that the only concern related to toxic contamination of natural ingredients. Studies on the graded effects of dietary factors were also bedevilled by the difficulty of quantifying intake of a nutrient, for example saturated fats, compared with the apparent simplicity of asking individuals how many cigarettes they smoked each day; how much easier it was to assess the impact in those who gave up smoking than in those who claimed they had changed their dietary habits.

Current Nutritional Issues

We will now have to come to terms with the complexity of nutrition, which spans from scientific areas as basic as the nutrient control of the molecular processes governing development to global policies and the future survival of some nation-states, for example Bangladesh.[8] Several examples from everyday life may serve to illustrate this.

Current Understanding of Coronary Heart Disease (CHD)

Although in the early 1960s Keys and his colleagues[9] clearly set out the three main risk factors for CHD, namely smoking, high blood pressure and an elevated blood cholesterol concentration, controversy has continued about the role of dietary factors in the development of CHD. Curiously, Keys' original data showed that smoking could be (1) extremely important for the development of heart disease, for example in Northern European countries such as Holland; (2) of only modest importance, as in the Mediterranean region; or (3) almost completely irrelevant, as in Japan. Thus in Northern Europe a middle-aged man smoking 20 cigarettes daily was over four times more at risk of a heart attack than non-smokers, but the risk was only 80 per cent higher in Italy or Crete. The Japanese, however, smoked as heavily as the Dutch and had the highest blood pressure in the world, but had a risk of heart disease which was less than one-tenth of the Northern European risk. Therefore, smoking was a risk factor only in the racially susceptible, or other environmental risk factors, such as diet, were important in promoting the impact of smoking or protecting the body from it. Several migrant studies soon established that racial susceptibility was not the explanation, which left other environmental risk factors. The only one then identified was the difference in serum cholesterol. It is therefore not surprising that Keys was so insistent that serum cholesterol was the principal issue. Once he had also established, in elegant physiological feeding studies in young men, that a specific range of saturated fatty acids induced the risk in cholesterol, the American Heart Foundation seemed totally justified in promoting preventive measures which included changing the type of fats eaten as well as stopping smoking. It took over 20 years and a national outcry over the National Advisory Committee on Nutrition Education in Britain Report[10] before the UK followed with specific and coherent proposals for dietary preventive measures.[11]

Keys' work was, in many ways, as plausible as the smoking analyses because animal studies showed that saturated fat feeding could induce coronary changes and patients with very high cholesterol levels, for what seemed like genetic reasons, were unusually susceptible to premature CHD. The poor response of cardiologists and general physicians to this argument in Europe stemmed not only from their training, which was dominated by seeing individual patients rather than considering public health issues, but also from the academic recognition that the pathophysiological processes were unknown and atherosclerosis seemed an insufficient explanation for CHD. Mitchell,[12] from the McMichael[13] school of iconoclasts, rightly pointed out that the clotting processes were likely to be of substantial importance and that concentrating only on the mechanism for arterial wall thickening was too naive. The importance of thrombosis is now recognized with marked dietary effects again being documented. We now also know that perhaps only half the variability in CHD is explained by the synergistic effects of smoking, high blood pressure and high cholesterol values.[14] Thus there are up to a dozen discrepancies in the saturated fatty acid-cholesterol hypothesis with, for example, the lower social classes being particularly susceptible despite having lower saturated fat intakes and lower serum cholesterol levels than the managerial classes who, despite their supposed stress, have a much lower risk of heart disease.[15] The current hypothesis of great interest and potentially capable of explaining many of the discrepancies is based on the protective role of vitamin E and vitamin C in preventing the oxidation of the circulating cholesterol and lipoproteins, thereby blocking the initiation of a free radical attack with selective uptake of oxidized fat into the arterial wall.[16] Dietary factors are also now being shown to modulate the levels of lipoprotein Lp(a) which is the most sensitive index of ischaemic risk.[17] It seems likely therefore that we will come to recognize that some individuals are indeed susceptible to CHD because they have the genetic make-up which makes them particularly responsive to individual saturated fatty acids, for example the C_{14} and C_{12} fatty acids, but even the risk of these effects on cholesterol levels can be modified by enhancing vegetable and fruit consumption to provide the 'protective factors' which, 50 or more years ago, were thought necessary simply to avoid scurvy or other trace deficiencies.

Diet and Cancer

Knowledge about the link between diet and the development of individual cancers is rapidly accumulating, but the mechanisms involved still elude us. Breast, stomach, colon, pancreatic, prostate and even lung cancers are increasingly linked to dietary factors, although the specific preventers and protectors remain uncertain. The concept of continuous free radical attack on the DNA of every cell in the body is now well accepted[18] and, despite the multiplicity of DNA repair mechanisms, new evidence suggests a huge increase in DNA damage with aging, this being particularly evident in smokers.[19] Epidemiologically, vegetable and fruit intake seems protective against stomach, breast and colon cancers; this may signify the role of vitamins E, C and other antioxidants in preventing DNA damage. The remarkably consistent findings, suggesting a protective effect of another vegetable-derived antioxidant, β-carotene, in smokers liable to develop lung cancer, is also noteworthy.[20] Other non-vitamin factors may also be involved, however, since phyto-oestrogens, for example, derived from soya, not only can have appreciable effects on the length of the menstrual cycle and other indices of sex hormone activity in women, but may also protect against breast cancer by blocking the promotional effects of naturally occurring oestrogens.[21] Our view of vitamin needs is also evolving since intakes of folic acid, which are sufficient for preventing anaemia and indeed maintaining plasma and red cell folate concentrations, may well be insufficient for maintaining the integrity of DNA.[22] Similarly, new evidence suggests that vitamin C helps to maintain the stability of DNA,[23] so that the need for these vitamins may in future be assessed on a completely different basis. Other nutrients may also affect sex hormone metabolism. Recent findings in animals suggest that both molybdenum and boron may interact to alter oestrogen metabolism by blocking the methylation of catechol oestrogens;[24] certainly excess molybdenum delays the onset of puberty in cattle, but there is no clear understanding of the detailed mechanism underlying the remarkable decrease in the age of onset of children's puberty during the twentieth century. There seems little doubt that changes in nutrition are somehow fundamentally involved, but we do not know whether it relates simply to accelerated growth rates in infancy and early childhood, to the earlier acquisition of a certain body size or fat mass, or to a steady decline in, for example, children's mineral-enriched intake of vegetables which also contain an array of biologically active molecules.

From this brief review, it seems clear that nutritional research will increasingly need to rely on chemists, molecular biologists and endocrinologists as well as epidemiologists if the role of diet in the development of some of the major health problems affecting affluent societies is to be unravelled.

Third World Nutrition

We have now moved to a view of nutrition where the problems seem to be very complex in our own society but very simple in the Third World. Those involved in development studies perceive that the big nutritional issues have already been identified and documented. The problem is then supposedly one of delivering the appropriate food to the vulnerable groups and relying on economic factors to solve the long-term problems of the purchasing power of the poor, their access to a varied diet and to the education necessary to improve their lot.

While there is much truth in this simplification, it should be approached with caution. For example, the principal nutritional problems of the Third World are perceived to be deficiencies of iodine, iron and vitamin A. These deficiencies are liable to affect literally billions of children and adults who often suffer permanent handicap.[25] With perhaps 90 per cent of Bangladesh's population short of iodine, the medical and social issues are huge. If, however, it is recognized that the primary problem is one of deficient soils in upper Bangladesh and Nepal exacerbated by flooding and deforestation, then the problem becomes even more complex. My feeling is that nutritionists not only have a role in promoting public awareness and government action; they must also continue to analyse nutritional problems carefully for discrepancies, since assumptions of the underlying nutritional condition may need to be challenged.

Some of these nutritional issues have enormous practical and political significance. Four examples may suffice to make the point. First, it is becoming apparent that iodine deficiency alone may not be the sole explanation of goitre and cretinism. Recently, Arthur and colleagues at the Rowett discovered that selenium is a fundamental component of the enzyme responsible for conversion of the circulating storage form of the thyroid hormone thyroxine to its metabolically active form, triiodothyronine, or T_3. The production of T_3 in the brain by the type II deiodinase enzyme also seems to be affected by selenium deficiency; the combination of selenium and iodine deficiency has much more profound effects than iodine deficiency alone.[26] Trials are now under way to test the importance of conjoint selenium and iodine supplementation, since administrators and politicians will clearly become disenchanted if their national programmes of iodination yield only modest success.

A second example of new discoveries comes from Golden's proposal that the infantile form of malnutrition, kwashiorkor, is yet another example of free radical damage, this time affecting the liver.[27] If this is true, as seems likely, then iron therapy for anaemic malnourished children may prove to be dangerous, as Golden points out, because cellular iron tends to promote free radical activity.

More problematic is Young's proposition that a normal adult's needs for essential amino acids have been seriously underestimated.[28] This disputed claim[29] could have serious repercussions, implying that the inclusion of an appreciable portion of animal protein in our diet to ensure an adequate intake of these essential components is sensible. Already the implications on a world basis are disquieting;[30] it is already well known that world cereal prices have depended on Russian purchases of excess American produce since the Soviet government had acted on the 1940s assumption that meat and milk were needed in abundance. Thus we have the curious spectacle of a crisis in food supplies to Russia and its neighbouring republics, whose populations have some of the highest rates of obesity in the world and where the real demand has been for cattle feeding to maintain the unnecessarily high intake of meat and milk. We forget too easily how major societal assumptions are locked into simple nutritional principles which have not been re-examined for half a century or more.

Finally, it may be appropriate to conclude on a personal note relating to world food supplies. Recently a group of nutritionists at the Rowett, including myself, was asked to propose a definition of chronic energy deficiency (CED) in adults, since those responsible for US aid sought to assess the need to provide food supplements for needy families. We recently refined the original definition[31] so that it now relies on body weight in relation to height alone.[32] To our astonishment, we discovered that, using simple criteria, 50 per cent of Indian adults had one of the three degrees of CED and that this rate was one of the worst in the world. With FAO

Table 2.1 Chronic energy deficiency (CED) in young adults aged 18–29 years in different parts of the world

	Men		*Women*	
Country	*Total*	*Grade III*	*Total*	*Grade III*
Asia				
China	11	1	13	1
India	50	9	49	11
Malaysia	11	–	15	–
Pakistan	48	–	40	–
Vietnam	28	1	29	2
Africa				
Togo	7	0	10	0
Benin	41	4	48	8
Ethiopia	49	5	58	6
Zimbabwe	15	1	12	1
Tunisia	5	0	5	1
South America				
Brazil	8	1	11	1

–, data not available. CED is defined on the basis of the same cut-off points of the body mass index (weight kg/height m^2) for men and women where Grade I = 17.0–18.4; Grade II = 16.0–16.9; and Grade III = <16.0. Data were provided to FAO by a large number of national agencies and experts.

support, we then analysed data from around the world and discovered that many of our common perceptions were wrong (see table 2.1). Further analyses showed that these grades of CED were predictive of illness and indeed death. In young women, the body mass index also predicted the likelihood of bearing low birth weight babies with all their well-recognized handicaps. Subsequent analyses show that we are not dealing with ethnic or racial differences but with a genuine problem of lifelong and adult nutrition. India therefore, while exporting food, has half its adult population, particularly in poor rural areas, more liable to illness and less able to sustain prolonged physical activity. In war-torn or drought-affected Africa, adult malnutrition is also a problem but in other parts of Africa the problems seem modest compared with those of Asia. Adult malnutrition has been neglected since World War II because the problem was considered simply as one of childhood malnutrition. On the basis of these analyses, our priorities have been misplaced for years and have led us to focus on the wrong parts of the world. If further analyses confirm these preliminary findings, then our aid and development programmes need to be completely revised.

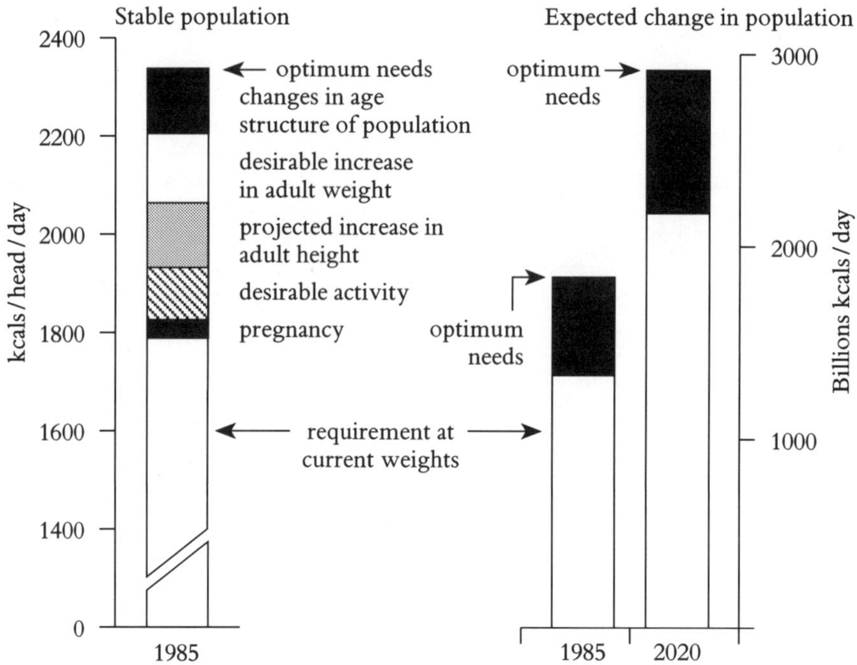

Figure 2.1 Projected food needs of the Indian population, 1985–2020.

In the long term, Asian food needs as depicted in figure 2.1 are also worrying. The figure shows my somewhat crude estimate of India's food needs based on a new approach to analysing population energy requirements.[33] Gopalan[34] has recently pointed out that soil erosion and degradation in India is so severe that present rates of food production are, in his opinion, unsustainable; he cites the likely development of widespread mineral deficiencies as the soil deteriorates and plants lose some of their nutritive value. If we add to these problems my own estimates of future population needs over the next 30 years, we begin to question some of our current complacency based on the capacity to apply scientific discoveries to the challenge. Recent global analyses suggest that salinity and erosion will lead to a loss of nearly 20 per cent of the world's agricultural land in the next decade.[35] If these FAO-based projections are correct, then the quantity of food available for sustaining societies will re-emerge as a top priority for the developing world as the issue of food quality is seen as ever more important in determining the public health of affluent societies.

NOTES

1 Corry Mann, H. C. (1926) 'Diet for boys during the school years', *Medical Research Council Special Report Series 105*, HMSO.

2 Petty, C. (1987) 'The impact of the newer knowledge of nutrition: nutrition science and nutrition policy, 1900–1939', Ph.D. Thesis, University of London.

3 Boyd Orr, J. (1936) *Food, Health and Income*, London, Macmillan.

4 Acheson, E. D. (1986) 'Food policy, nutrition and government', *Proceedings of the Nutrition Society* 45, 131–8.

5 Cannon, G. (1992) *Food and Health: the experts agree*, London, Consumers' Association.

6 Peto, R., Lopez, A. D., Boreham, J., Thun, M. and Heath, C. (1992) 'Mortality from tobacco in developed countries: indirect estimation from national vital statistics', *Lancet* 339, 1268–78.

7 Taylor, P. (1984) *Smoke Ring: the politics of tobacco*, London, The Bodley Head.

8 James, W. P. T. and Ralph, A. (1993) 'Nutrition and health tomorrow', in P. Leathwood, M. Horisberger and W. P. T. James (eds) *For a Better Nutrition in the 21st Century*, Nestlé Nutrition Workshop Series, Vol. 27, New York, Nestec Ltd, Vevey/Raven Press Ltd.

9 Keys, A. (1980) *Seven Countries: a multivariate analysis of death and coronary heart disease*, London, Harvard University Press.

10 National Advisory Committee on Nutrition Education in Britain (1983) Proposals for nutritional guidelines for health education in Britain, London, Health Education Council.

11 Department of Health and Social Security (1984) Diet and cardiovascular disease. Committee on medical aspects of food policy, London, HMSO.

12 Mitchell, J. R. A. (1984) 'What constitutes evidence on the dietary prevention of coronary heart disease? Cosy beliefs or harsh facts', *International Journal of Cardiology* 5, 287–98.

13 McMichael, J. (1976) 'Prevention of Coronary Heart Disease' (Letter), *Lancet* ii, 569.

14 Marmot, M. G., Shipley, M. J. and Rose, G. (1984) 'Inequalities in death – specific explanations of a general pattern?', *Lancet* i, 1003–6.

15 James, W. P. T., Duthie, G. G. and Wahle, K. W. J. (1989) 'The Mediterranean diet: protective or simply non-toxic?', *European Journal of Clinical Nutrition* 43 (Suppl. 2), 31–41.

16 Duthie, G. G., Wahle, K. W. J. and James, W. P. T. (1989) 'Oxidants, antioxidants and cardiovascular disease', *Nutrition Research Reviews* 2, 51–62.

17 MBewu, A. D. and Durrington, P. N. (1990) 'Lipoprotein (a): structural properties and possible involvement in thrombogenesis and atherogenesis', *Atherosclerosis* 85, 1–14.

18 Ames, B. N. (1989) 'Endogenous DNA damage as related to cancer and aging', *Mutation Research* 214, 41–6.

19 Cole, J., Waugh, A. P. W., Bear, D. M., Salar-Trepat, M., Stephens, G. and Green, M. H. L. (1991) 'Hprt mutant frequencies in circulating lymphocytes: population studies using normal donors, exposed groups and cancer-prone syndromes', in B. L. Gledhill and F. Mauro, *New Horizons in Biological Dosimetry*, Chichester, Wiley-Liss Inc.

20 Willett, W. (1990) 'Nutritional epidemiology', *Monographs in Epidemiology and Biostatistics*, Vol. 15, New York, Oxford University Press.
21 Lee, H. P., Gourley, L., Duffy, S. W., Esteve, J., Lee, J. and Day, N. E. (1991) 'Dietary effects on breast cancer risk in Singapore', *Lancet* 337, 1197–1200.
22 MacGregor, J. T. (1989) 'Dietary factors affecting spontaneous chromosomal damage in man', in M. W. Pariza, H. U. Aeschbacher, J. S. Felton and S. Sato (eds) *Mutagens and Carcinogens in the Diet*, New York, Wiley-Liss, pp. 139–53.
23 Fraga, C. G., Motchnik, P. A., Shigenaga, M. K., Helbock, H. J. and Jacob, R. A. (1991) 'Ascorbic and protects against endogenous oxidative DNA damage in human sperm', *Proceeding of the National Academy of Sciences USA* 88, 11003–6.
24 Beattie, J. H. and Weersink, E. (1991) 'Borate and molybdate inhibition of catechol estrogen and pyrocatechol methylation by catechol-o-methyl transferase', *Journal of Inorganic Chemistry* 46, 153–60.
25 World Health Organization (1990) 'Diet, nutrition and the prevention of chronic diseases', *Technical Report Series* 797, Geneva.
26 Arthur, J. R. (1991) 'The role of selenium in thyroid hormone metabolism', *Canadian Journal of Physiology and Pharmacology* 69, 1648–52.
27 Golden, M. H. N. and Ramdath, D. D. (1987) 'Free radicals in the pathogenesis of kwashiorkor', *Proceedings of the Nutrition Society* 46, 53–68.
28 Young, V., Bier, D. M. and Pellet, P. L. (1989) 'A theoretical basis for increasing current estimates of the amino acid requirements in adult man with experimental support', *American Journal of Clinical Nutrition* 50, 80–92.
29 Millward, D. J. and Rivers, J. (1988) 'The nutritional role of indispensable amino acids and the metabolic basis for their requirements', *European Journal of Clinical Nutrition* 42, 367–93.
30 Kazno, H. (1991) 'Current world supplies of and requirements for essential amino acids', *Food and Nutrition Bulletin* 13, 29–39.
31 James, W. P. T., Ferro-Luzzi, A. and Waterlow, J. C. (1988) 'Definition of chronic energy deficiency in adults', *European Journal of Clinical Nutrition* 42, 969–81.
32 Ferro-Luzzi, A., Sette, S., Franklin, J. and James, W. P. T. (1992) 'A simplified approach of assessing chronic energy deficiency', *European Journal of Clinical Nutrition* 46, 173–86.
33 James, W. P. T. and Schofield, E. C. (1990) *Human Energy Requirements*, Oxford, Oxford Medical Publications.
34 Gopalan, C. (1991) 'Challenges and frontiers in nutrition in Asia', *Proceedings of the 6th Asian Congress of Nutrition*, Kuala Lumpur, 1–20.
35 *Economist*, April 1991.

3

The Evolution of Diets for Western Diseases

A. Stewart Truswell

From around 1950 with recovery from World War II, research in human nutrition changed direction in the affluent countries from a search for new deficiency diseases to a slow realization that the major degenerative diseases of older life might be at least partly determined by something as humble, as domestic, as enjoyable as the foods we eat habitually. By now there is an unwieldy mass of evidence from different disciplines with which we can put together very incomplete pictures of the complex involvement of diet in the causation and/or treatment of coronary heart artery disease, diabetes and high blood pressure.

Development of each of these concepts has been – and still is – a hard journey with false trails, skirmishes, wasted resources, confused languages and no clear end. Many hypotheses arise but only the fittest survive and they are changed in the process. The reason for this complex, rather wasteful process is that elucidation of the contributions of diet to these multifactorial diseases has to depend on accumulation of different types of indirect evidence.

Coronary Heart Disease

Although Aschoff first drew attention to the high content of cholesterol in atheromatous aortas in 1906,[1] it was not until 1950 that the relationship between the plasma cholesterol level and coronary heart disease (CHD) began to be recognized. Until then it had been highly controversial. Demonstration of higher plasma cholesterol in CHD than controls required the adoption of statistical methods, age standardization and appropriate controls. This association in case-control (retrospective) studies within a community was confirmed in comparisons between different communities by

Ancel Keys and collaborators[2] and subsequently in the findings of prospective (cohort) studies, first in Framingham, Massachusetts.[3] The relationship of plasma (total) cholesterol and CHD was accepted as a *causal* factor (among multiple factors) by a World Health Organization (WHO) Expert Committee in 1982 and by the US National Institutes of Health Consensus Development Conference in 1985.

This means that the quest for dietary factors in CHD can be approached by the shorter route of examining how they affect plasma cholesterol concentration.

There are, however, three main classes of lipids in the blood and another class, the triglycerides (measured after fasting, because a fatty meal raises the level) were reported to be associated with CHD in retrospective studies. Multivariate analyses, with computers, to allow for interrelationships with other risk factors, have not however shown an independent relationship of triglycerides with CHD. Plasma triglycerides are more variable from day to day than cholesterol; they fall after moderate exercise.

Cholesterol is carried in the plasma combined with special lipoproteins. Most is carried on low-density lipoproteins (LDL, separable by their low density in a very fast centrifuge). It is the LDL-cholesterol that is responsible for the association of total plasma cholesterol with CHD. High-density lipoproteins (HDL) were first reported negatively associated with CHD but this protective relationship was not generally recognized until the mid-1970s, after analysis of HDLs in prospective studies.

Dietary Cholesterol

By feeding cholesterol Anitschkow in St Petersburg produced fatty accumulations in rabbits' arteries, resembling atherosclerosis as early as 1913, but this did not happen in rats and was considered a laboratory curiosity until the early 1950s. In man, Ancel Keys found the effect of dietary cholesterol on plasma cholesterol to be negligible.[4] Over 100 sets of human feeding experiments since then have shown variable responses, on average small increases of plasma cholesterol; some individuals are responders, some not. Part of the cholesterol in our plasma is synthesized in the liver from acetate; absorption of ingested cholesterol is poor. When more (exogenous) cholesterol is eaten endogenous synthesis tends to be switched off.

Dietary Total Fat

The surprising phenomenon that (total) fat has more effect in raising plasma cholesterol than dietary cholesterol was discovered around 1950.[5] Falls of cholesterol had been noticed in patients treated for hypertension with the rice-fruit diet (very low in fat).[6] This gave the first real hope of 'prediction and possible prevention of coronary disease' and was soon supported by cross-sectional epidemiological studies made by Keys and collaborators.[7]

Saturated, Monounsaturated and Polyunsaturated Fats

The next discovery, in 1956, was that dietary fats do not all have the same effect on plasma (LDL) cholesterol; saturated fatty acids raise cholesterol, polyunsaturated lower cholesterol and monounsaturated fatty acids have an intermediate effect.[8] This was demonstrated in metabolically normal subjects, e.g. chronic schizophrenics, housed in metabolic units where their dietary fats were exchanged periodically with a series of mixtures of natural edible fats and oils. The predominant polyunsaturated fatty acid here is linoleic acid (18:2) belonging to the omega-6 family. In the classic seven country (11 community) prospective study the incidence of CHD could be correlated with the community's saturated fat intake, not with its total fat intake.[9] Diets on the principle of reduced saturated and total fat and cholesterol and moderately increased polyunsaturated fat have been used in most of the prevention trials of CHD and form a major part of dietary guidelines for health for Western countries.

Diets low in saturated fats with increased polyunsaturated (omega-6) fats appear to reduce the tendency to thrombosis and, in animals, also reduce the susceptibility of the heart to dangerous rhythm disturbances when its blood supply is reduced.

Fish Oils

Fish body oils contain important amounts of eicosapentaenoic acid (20:5, ω-3), precursor of thromboxane TxA_3 which does not have the aggregatory effect on platelets of the usual TxA_2 (derived from arachidonic acid). Greenland Eskimos eat a high (marine) fat diet and have plasma cholesterols in the middle range but little cardiovascular disease. Moderate intakes of fish appear to confer some protection against CHD in some other populations (but not all). Fish-oil polyunsaturated fatty acids reduce plasma triglycerides more but cholesterol less than omega-6 polyunsaturated fats. Expert committees, while encouraging moderate intake of fish, do not advise the use of concentrated fish-oil supplements except under medical supervision.

Individual Fatty Acids

Calculations made in the late 1950s and 1960s that saturated fats raise plasma cholesterol, polyunsaturated have half as strong a lowering effect and monounsaturated are neutral have to be modified in the light of human experiments in the late 1980s.

Monounsaturated fatty acids, principally oleic (18:1), now appear to be cholesterol-lowering[10] though this probably depends on the linoleic acid content of the test diets. Though reduction of LDL-cholesterol tends to be less than with linoleic acid (omega-6 polyunsaturated), monounsaturated fats seem less liable to reduce HDL-cholesterol (a presumably undesirable effect). This re-evaluation fits with the very low incidence of coronary disease among Cretans who consume quite large amounts of fat as olive oil (predominantly monounsaturated).

Stearic acid (18:0) though saturated does not raise cholesterol in the form of mixtures of natural fats. However in semisynthetic fats stearic acid has a moderate cholesterol-raising effect, perhaps because of a different arrangement of fatty acids on the dietary triglycerides. While it can thus be regarded as neutral in its atherogenic effect (i.e. on LDL-cholesterol), there is evidence that stearic acid tends to promote thrombosis.

As to the other common saturated fatty acids, recent work in humans, supported by tests with precisely formulated diets in primates, supports observations in the 1960s that palmitic acid (16:0) does not raise cholesterol as much as myristic (14:0) and lauric (12:0) acids do. Palmitic is the most abundant saturated fatty acid in edible fats and oils.

Natural unsaturated fatty acids normally have double bonds in the *cis*-configuration (bent shape). *Trans*-fatty acids (straight shape), about 5 per cent of the fatty acids in modern diets, are a by-product when polyunsaturated fats are hardened by hydrogenation in making margarines. Small amounts are formed naturally by microbial hydrogenation in ruminants and go into beef, lamb and milk fat. The main *trans*-fatty acid is *trans*-18:1 (the stereoisomer of oleic acid), called elaidic. Trans-fatty acids raise LDL-cholesterol and may also lower HDL-cholesterol.[11] The UK Committee on Medical Aspects of Food Policy recommends that trans-fatty acids be regarded as equivalent to saturated fatty acids for the purposes of preventing CHD.

Instead of lumping all dietary saturated fatty acids together we should take account of their different cholesterol-elevating effects. In descending order, this appears to be (most cholesterol-elevating) myristic (14:0), lauric (12:0), palmitic (16:0), trans-monounsaturated (18:1trans) and stearic (18:0) (least cholesterol-elevating).

Dietary Protein

In humans plasma cholesterol level is low in the kwashiorkor form of protein-energy malnutrition[12] but when protein and amino acid requirements are met most investigators have reported no convincing effect of dietary protein, quantity or quality, with one exception. Exchange of soy protein for casein (with dietary fat and fibre constant) leads to lower plasma cholesterol in rabbits; in man this soy protein effect has been variable. It seems to be more reproducible in people with hypercholesterolaemia and soy protein has to be more than half the protein intake.

Pursuing different hypotheses, supplements of individual pure amino acids have been tried in man: methionine, leucine, taurine, glutamic acid and histidine, all with no effect on plasma cholesterol.

A claim that whole milk does not raise plasma cholesterol because the effect of the cream is neutralized by a cholesterol-lowering property of the aqueous phase of milk has not be confirmed.

Carbohydrates

A high carbohydrate diet is a low fat diet since people's total protein intake (under normal conditions) is always near 10 to 15 per cent of calories. Populations that consume high (total) carbohydrate diets have a low incidence of CHD and in prospective studies individuals with higher carbohydrate intake have also had a lower incidence of CHD.

There are three main types of dietary carbohydrate: sugars, starches and non-starch polysaccharides (dietary fibre). The hypothesis that sugar (sucrose) is the main cause of CHD rested principally on associations of sucrose consumption and CHD between countries and with time in the UK. It had a major influence on policy in Britain for 20 years.[13] In other affluent countries the sugar hypothesis did not displace preventive action to reduce saturated fat intake and CHD incidence started to decline from the mid-1960s, although in the UK CHD incidence remained static until 1984 brought better official guidance. Sugar does not satisfy the criteria for incriminating a dietary component in causation of CHD[14, 15] and is not now included in authoritative recommendations.

If carbohydrate intake is increased but calories remain constant, plasma cholesterol falls because the amount of fat in the diet has gone down. Plasma triglycerides increase (only the fasting concentration) but may not stay high in the long term.

Trowell proposed that dietary fibre could protect against CHD in 1972 as part of the dietary fibre hypothesis.[16] He pointed out that CHD incidence in Britain had varied over time with the intake of wheat fibre. The most obvious *direct* mechanism for such an effect is by reduction of plasma LDL-cholesterol, by interference with sterol metabolism, in the gut, since dietary fibre is indigestible and not absorbable as such. The hypothesis stimulated much research, including as many as 200 reported feeding experiments with groups of human subjects. It is now clear that wheat fibre and other types of insoluble fibre do not directly lower plasma cholesterol but other types – 'soluble' or viscous food fibres in pectin, oat bran, psyllium and guar can.[17] A high fibre intake also has *indirect* effects, either because high fibre foods are low in fat and displace fat in the diet, or because of associated protective substances in some vegetable foods.

Overweight and Obesity

Obesity is an inconsistent and largely indirect risk factor for CHD. People who are overweight or obese have increased risk of diabetes and tend to have higher LDL-cholesterol and blood pressure, and lower HDL-cholesterol, but if these other risk factors are held constant in multifactorial analysis much epidemiological data indicate that obesity makes only a small independent contribution to the risk of CHD.[18] In the Seven Country Study neither body weight nor skinfold thickness helped to explain the differences in CHD between the populations.[9] Risk of CHD from overweight is greater in younger adults and when it develops rapidly and where it is central (high waist/hip ratio). In the Framingham prospective study, at 12 years' follow-up, obesity was only associated with increased risk of angina pectoris and sudden death in men, not myocardial infarction and not CHD in women.[19] After 26 years' follow-up, it had become clear that increasing relative weight was an independent risk factor for CHD in men and women, though less powerful than serum cholesterol.

Alcohol

Pathologists have long noticed absence of atheroma in alcoholics. Klatsky reported in 1974 an excess of teetotallers in a group of Americans with a first myocardial infarct.[20] By now this has been confirmed in 17 prospective studies in eight different countries. The Honolulu Heart Study has been particularly informative because of its substantial proportion of lifetime abstainers. Here the graph of total mortality against alcohol intake was noted to be U-shaped and this curve has been found in other studies. Small and moderate alcohol intake is associated with protection from coronary heart disease (relative risk about 0.7) but above two or three drinks a day the incidence of other cardiovascular diseases, including hypertension and haemorrhagic stroke, starts to increase. There are two mechanisms to explain the protective effect: increased concentration of HDL-cholesterol (HDL_2, HDL_3 and apolipoproteins AI and AII) repeatedly demonstrated since the 1970s, and (a new hypothesis) reduced aggregation of platelets.

Coffee

In a large retrospective study in Boston it was found that patients surviving a myocardial infarct had consumed more coffee than matched controls.[21]

This could not be explained by association with other risk factors. However, in the major prospective studies amount of coffee consumed did not come out as a risk factor and the Royal College of Physicians working party (1976) concluded: 'There is at present no firm evidence that coffee drinking is a factor in the development of . . . CHD'.[18] Interest was reawakened in the 1980s by the puzzling association of coffee consumption with higher plasma cholesterols in some (Scandinavian) countries but not others. It was originally assumed that caffeine would be the active ingredient but in direct experiments cholesterol is no higher on standard coffee than decaffeinated. In Tromsø workers discovered that boiled coffee raises plasma cholesterol but filtered coffee does not.[22] Zock et al.[23] report a cholesterol-lowering fraction in the tiny lipid phase of boiled coffee. At the epidemiological level a prospective study of Johns Hopkins medical students showed that, while original coffee consumption was not related to subsequent CHD, people change this habit over time and the most recent records of coffee intake had a positive association with CHD.[24]

Soft and Hard Water

The report of higher death rate from *all* cardiovascular diseases in communities with soft water[25] rests on comparisons between different towns. Much of the research to try to explain and confirm the hypothesis has been done in Britain. The infant death rate is also inversely related to water calcium in Britain. The towns with soft water are mostly in the north of England and Scotland while the communities drinking hard water are in the more prosperous south-east of England. There are therefore a number of other environmental and sociological differences between these communities. In some other countries opposite findings have been documented and in Britain Birmingham is a major exception; its large population received soft water but has a relatively low CHD mortality. No physiological mechanism has yet been isolated, so the water hypothesis cannot be tested experimentally. In the British Regional Heart Study, comparing many variables in 253 British towns, multifactorial analysis indicated that water calcium explains 10–15 per cent of differences in mortality from CHD and stroke, the rest being attributable to rainfall, temperature, percentage of manual workers and car ownership.[26] Towns which were artificially softening their naturally hard water supply did not seem to have higher cardiovascular mortality than matched towns.

Free Oxygen Radicals and Antioxidants

The newest hypothesis might also help to explain some of the variations in CHD between different parts of Britain. Experimental pathology research shows that the characteristic foam cells of atheroma result from uptake of LDL by blood monocytes and tissue macrophages (the same cell in a different place) in the arterial wall but this happens very slowly unless the lipids of LDL are partly oxidized. We have less idea about which are the sources of free oxygen radicals than we have of protective substances that could be augmented. These are the antioxidant nutrients, fat-soluble vitamin E and β-carotene and water-soluble vitamin C.

Supportive evidence for this hypothesis comes from epidemiological studies which show an inverse correlation of plasma vitamin E and CHD between communities, and within a Scottish community an inverse association between plasma vitamin E and angina (still significant after adjustment for other risk factors).

None of this is proof that present differences in intake of antioxidant nutrients are important determinants of the incidence of CHD or (a somewhat different question) whether unusually large intakes of one or more of these antioxidants from special diets or supplements can give worthwhile protection. Useful answers will come from controlled prevention trials, such as the ß-carotene trials under way in the United States and some other countries. A lot of research is now being done on different aspects of this hypothesis. Clear results will probably take years. In the meantime, popularizers of science have, as usual, jumped the gun and are advising that we eat more vegetables and fruits. As long as we continue reducing saturated fat intake this can do no harm and may do good.

Changing Mortality Rates

In the last 30 years age-standardized deaths from CHD have declined by more than 60 per cent in the USA, Australia and Canada and by somewhat smaller amounts in New Zealand, Switzerland, Finland, Belgium and Israel. Total (all causes) mortality has declined too in these countries. By contrast, the countries of Eastern Europe, for example Hungary, Poland, the Czech and Slovak Republics, have suffered large increases in coronary deaths, accompanied by rises in total mortality. In an intermediate group of countries changes in coronary mortality have been small or late, for example Sweden, Denmark, Ireland, England and Wales, Scotland and Northern Ireland. Exact rank order in this league table depends to some extent on the period compared but there is no longer any doubt about the big picture. Those who have examined the changes in contrasting countries have concluded that dietary change appears to have been the most consistent variable in lifestyle, notably an increase in omega-6 polyunsaturated fatty acid consumption in the countries with falling mortality and an increase in animal fat in the countries with rising coronary and total mortality. In England and Wales, CHD mortality started to move downwards from about 1977, which coincides with the start of an increase in the polyunsaturated/saturated fatty acid ratio in the average household diet. Oliver's group in Edinburgh[27] found significant inverse and progressive relations between adipose-tissue linoleic acid (18:2) and risk of CHD in a population-based case-control study. Four other case-control studies have had similar findings. Doubtless less smoking and better medical and surgical management have also played a role, but these other improvements have been much the same across all western countries.

Diabetic Diets

It is commonly assumed that there is one diabetic diet, with fine tuning for the individual's likes and dislikes as well as pocket. But at any one time there are different nutritional principles and interpretations placed on foods between diabetic clinics, even within the same country. There is also a gap between the diabetic diet on paper and the diabetic diet actually eaten. Perhaps the most fascinating story is how diets prescribed for treatment of diabetes have changed since the early 1900s (see table 3.1).

Before the discovery of insulin the only question for insulin-dependent diabetes (i.e. in younger adults) was how many weeks or months the patient survived. Osler, in his textbook of medicine (1913),[28] placed the patient on a non-carbohydrate diet 'consisting of meat, eggs, butter, olive oil, leafy vegetables and whiskey'. Urine sugar decreased greatly and if it disappeared small amounts of starch could be added to the diet, 20 or 50 g until the glycosuria reappeared. If control was difficult a 'hunger day' could be tried. An alternative diet at that time (interesting because of a modern revival of its named ingredient) was von Noorden's oatmeal diet: 250 g of oatmeal, mixed with the same amount of butter and the whites of 7 eggs, cooked together and taken in portions during the day with black coffee, tea or whiskey.[28] A third regime, the Allen diet, was very low in calories provided as protein and fat and led to severe loss of weight and strength, but Allen claimed his patients survived longer. These diets were very complicated; they required obsessional dietary management, regular weighing and daily analysis of sugar and nitrogen in the urine. Only about 5 per cent of calories came from carbohydrates and 75 to 80 per cent from fat.

When insulin came into use from 1922 it was at first in short supply and doctors were cautious in using it. The very low carbohydrate, very high fat diets were continued, quite reasonably, for the first few years of the insulin era. In the 1930 edition of Price's textbook of medicine[29] for example, a typical dietary prescription had 15 per cent calories from carbohydrate and 70 per cent from fat. This was used at St Bartholomew's Hospital in London, and at the London Hospital, the proportions were the same.

Table 3.1 Diabetic diets, 1900–90

Year	*Prescribed diet*
1900–25	Fasting (Allen diet), 5% carbohydrate, 75–80% fat
1922	Insulin
1930	Very low carbohydrate, e.g. 30%, and 70% fat
1940–50	Low all carbohydrate e.g. 30%, and 50% fat
1970	Round 40% carbohydrate Sugar prohibited Insulin or oral drugs emphasized
1980	50–60% carbohydrate, as 'complex' carbohydrate A little sugar Reduction in fat
1990	50–60% carbohydrate: emphasis on low glycaemic index foods Low saturated fat Overweight often the biggest challenge

In the 1940s and 1950s, the carbohydrate allowance had come up to 25 to 30 per cent in British diabetic diets, i.e., the fat was 50–55 per cent, and carbohydrate exchange lists were used, for example R. D. Lawrence's 'black lines'.[30] There appears to have been little questioning of the theoretical basis that carbohydrates were bad for diabetics. But with insulin, patients could be allowed to eat a diet somewhat nearer to what their non-diabetic family members were eating.

By around 1970, different types of insulin complicated the physician's work. Many patients complied poorly and even if obese non-insulin-dependent diabetics (NIDDs) did not manage to eat less, their glucose metabolism could now be controlled with the new oral hypoglycaemic drugs. Drugs were easier for doctors to understand and quicker to prescribe than diets, and doctors were encouraged by the pharmaceutical companies. In a major North American textbook diets were hardly mentioned.[31]

Dietitians in Britain at this time were instructing patients to eat around 40 per cent of their energy as carbohydrate but prohibition of sucrose was now the major message. This was not based on any convincing experimental data but probably reflected the fashionable hypothesis of that period – that sucrose was the main cause of many diseases of Western adults.

Since about the mid-1970s there has been a slow revolution of thinking about diabetic diets and an important accumulation of human experimental data from acute test meal studies and a few longer-term trials.

1 Oral hypoglycaemic drugs may predispose to heart disease in diabetics. Although dietary change means more work for health professionals and for patients, it may be safer.

2 Diabetics in developed countries no longer die of diabetic ketoacidosis. Their major causes of death are arterial diseases, especially coronary heart disease. Diabetics tend to have higher plasma cholesterols than non-diabetics. Diabetic diets, in lowering the per cent energy from carbohydrate, have been *high fat* diets and in western countries the fat is mainly saturated. Asian diabetics, though continuing to eat diets higher in carbohydrate than western diabetic patients, appear to have fewer complications, especially atherosclerotic, like coronary heart disease.

Back in 1928 Joslin, America's leading diabetic specialist, wondered whether 'the prevalence of arteriosclerosis in diabetes is to be attributed to the high fat diets we have prescribed'.[32] He proposed limiting eggs and thought that this therapeutic procedure should not take long for experimental investigation!

3 As early as 1936, Himsworth (later Sir Harold) reported that a high carbohydrate diet *improves* the glucose tolerance test of healthy individuals.[33] Cautiously and with trepidation, a series of diabetologists tested the effect of higher carbohydrate diets on diabetics in controlled trials. In general, glucose status was no worse than on traditional diets and plasma cholesterol fell. Apart from an exceptional trial in 1938 which was overlooked, the trials of high carbohydrate diets were reported from 1958, through the 1960s and into the 1970s. The first of these investigators were lone voices crying in the wilderness but, during the 1970s, the accumulating evidence that low carbohydrate diets were no longer appropriate, impressed an increasing number of physicians. Authoritative committees in Britain, the USA and elsewhere all now recommend relatively high carbohydrate diets as the standard management for diabetes. There remains, however, a conservative minority and a high *mono*unsaturated fat diet compared well with a high carbohydrate diet in one study.

4 Hugh Trowell[34] suggested that dietary fibre might protect genetically susceptible humans from the development of diabetes on high starch diets – particularly wheat fibre. Mortality from diabetes declined when the extraction rate of flour was increased in the British diet during World War II (there were, of course, many other national changes). The first demonstration that a concentrated fibre supplement can improve glucose metabolism

in diabetes was by Jenkins et al. from Oxford: a large dose of guar gum reduced urinary glucose.[35] Guar is a viscous, soluble type of 'fibre', like pectin and some of the fibre in legumes. These reduce the rise of blood glucose after a meal. Insoluble types of fibre such as wheat bran do not do this.

5 Most fibre is carbohydrate and some of the successful high carbohydrate diets for diabetes have been high in fibre, but guar is not a natural food and high fibre diets have been rather unpalatable. The enthusiasm for high fibre diets of the 1970s and early 1980s has waned and been replaced by a new concept that differences in the digestibility of starch have more impact. Starches in different foods do not produce the same rise of blood sugar; they vary quite considerably in *glycaemic index*. Many of the starchy staples of western diets like bread and potatoes have a high glycaemic index: the increase of blood glucose above fasting after the amount of the food that contains a standard weight of carbohydrate is nearly as high as after the same weight of glucose. In other foods, such as pasta, legumes, oatmeal and whole grains, the starch takes longer to digest and there is a smaller rise of the blood glucose.

Until recently, designers of diabetic diets assumed that all carbohydrates produce the same rise of blood glucose after they were eaten, provided that the dose of carbohydrate was the same, except that table sugar (sucrose) would give a higher level. Elaborate carbohydrate exchange lists were published, for example 1 orange = a glass of milk = 2/3 a thin slice of bread. These foods don't have the same effect on blood glucose but this has only been tested in human experiments from about 1980. Glycaemic index can be affected by a food's processing or cooking method, which also cuts across traditional exchange lists. Fat in a meal delays gastric emptying and fat-rich foods can have a low glycaemic index but not be good for diabetics. Glycaemic indices of foods must therefore be compared at equal fat intake levels.

A few intermediate term trials have now been carried out to test the practical value of glycaemic index. In the first of these in adults by Brand et al.,[36] palatable combinations of low glycaemic foods gave significantly better diabetic control in patients with non-insulin-dependent diabetes (NIDDM) in a 3-month/3-month crossover trial.

6 Because some starchy foods have a high glycaemic index and some sugars have low glycaemic index, terms like 'complex' and 'simple' carbohydrates now have little use in planning diabetic diets. For sucrose the wheel has almost come full circle. Its glycaemic index is 60, which is to be expected since it is a disaccharide made of equal parts glucose (glycaemic index 100) and fructose (glycaemic index 20, hence the low glycaemic index of many fruits). This means that sucrose is not the worst food a diabetic can eat. Indeed, Brand has shown that addition of sucrose to high glycaemic index processed starchy foods lowers their glycaemic index.

7 Lastly, most diabetic patients have the non-insulin-dependent (NID) type of diabetes. Most NID diabetics are overweight or obese. When overweight NID diabetics manage to lose weight their diabetes improves considerably. This can be observed even when weight loss has been modest and before the patient reaches a normal weight for height. However, the majority of overweight diabetics do not manage to lose much body weight or keep it off. The overwhelming objective in their dietary treatment is to reduce weight by combining a low-calorie diet with increased exercise (which improves sensitivity to insulin). In diabetic research and service there has been too little money and resources put into understanding and treating overweight and obesity.

Prevention

This understanding we have slowly gained about diets for treating symptomatic diabetes is applicable to the larger numbers of people with prediabetes or a strong family history, for whom up to now there has been very little available for prophylaxis. Epidemiological data indicate that high fat and calorie intakes, not high carbohydrate or sugar, are associated with non-insulin-dependent diabetes.

Diet and Blood Pressure

The idea that diet can influence blood pressure originates in two sets of observations. One is that the prevalence of hypertension, high blood pressure, varies greatly between different communities. It has to be age-standardized because where hypertension is common, average blood pressure goes up with age; it also depends on the cut-off levels for diagnosis and the method used for measurement. In middle-aged adults, the prevalence has varied between 0 per cent and 40 per cent. It does not seem to be related to the stresses of modern life since it can occur in even very remote communities. Secondly, high blood pressures have been noted to fall with certain changes in diet.

Salt: Sodium Chloride

Salt is the best known of the dietary factors affecting blood pressure. It has been hypothesized for the longest time; there is abundant epidemiological and experimental data and there has also been lively controversy. Ambard and Beaujard first suggested that salt was a cause of raised blood pressure in 1904.[37] Then Allen in 1922 documented reduction of blood pressure by salt restriction.[38] Kempner was responsible for the second wave of salt restriction 25 years later.[6] His rice-fruit diet lowered blood pressure in 65 per cent of his patients. Both these pioneers were unpopular and had little following. Dole and co-workers[39] demonstrated that the effect of the rice-fruit diet was due to its very low salt content (only 150 mg of sodium per day). One of this group, Lewis Dahl built up the salt hypothesis, with careful therapeutic studies, a practical low salt diet and development of a rat model. He was the first to claim that prevalence of hypertension in selected countries correlated with their average daily salt intake. About 20 remote communities have been reported that do not (or did not) suffer from hypertension; their mean blood pressure doesn't rise with age: they do not have access to salt (or did not, because several of these communities now have salt and experience high blood pressure).

Evidence for the salt hypothesis is by now considerable.

1 Thiazide and similar diuretics lower blood pressure. They do so by producing a negative sodium balance.
2 Meta-analysis of observational data between different communities. In 24 communities (47,000 people) on average, systolic blood pressure is 5 mm higher at age 17 and 10 mm Hg higher at 65 years for 100 mmol difference in sodium intake.
3 Meta-analysis of observational data within populations. There is a significant trend but the slopes of the regression lines are reduced because of the large day-to-day variation in 24-hour sodium intake within individuals.
4 Meta-analysis of 78 controlled trials of salt reduction. It is clear that restriction of salt to somewhere below 100 mmol sodium per day will usually lower blood pressure in people with hypertension. It is sometimes sufficient but often needs to be supplemented with medication. Blood pressure usually falls in normotensive people, but not in a minority. It is sodium chloride, not other sodium salts like bicarbonate, that is related to blood pressure.

The bigger and more difficult question is whether the salt consumption of most people in most countries – about 10 times the nutrition requirement and 20 times what breast feeding supplies to infants – can be regarded as a major cause or conditioning factor of essential hypertension. In a community eating more than 100 mmol of sodium/day, who gets hypertension is not directly related to salt intake. There must be some who are sensitive and more who are not. Salt sensitivity increases with age and is commoner in blacks than whites. Probable mechanisms involved in salt sensitivity are reductions in the ability to transport sodium out of cells or failure to increase renal blood flow and aldosterone secretion after a high intake of sodium.

Some authoritative committees now accept that the evidence is sufficiently persuasive (and the health risks of reducing salt intake sufficiently slight) to recommend to the general public a target of sodium intake below 100 mmol/day (6 g sodium chloride). In Japan, which used to have very high prevalences of hypertension, these have been declining rapidly, along with mortality from strokes since the Ministry of Health advised reduction of salt to 10 g/day. When Dahl first compared different countries in 1961, Japan (main island) had over 20 per cent prevalence of hypertension, but in the recent Intersalt study, rates in three Japanese cities were only 11 per cent.

Potassium

Potassium is in several ways an antagonist to sodium. Administration of potassium for example increases urinary sodium excretion. In modern technological society, our foods have had sodium added during processing and cooking; against this, some of their original potassium may be refined or dissolved out.

The sodium/potassium ratio for wheat changes from $\frac{1}{100}$ to 5.0.

Wholemeal wheat flour	contains sodium 3,	potassium 360 mg/100 g
White wheat flour	contains sodium 3,	potassium 130 mg/100 g
Wholemeal wheat bread	contains sodium 540,	potassium 220 mg/100 g
White wheaten bread	contains sodium 540,	potassium 100 mg/100 g

Addison in Canada,[40] then Priddle,[41] reported reduction of blood pressure in hypertensive cases with different salts of potassium over 60 years ago, and McQuarrie[42] reported reduction of blood pressure in children by potassium chloride (KCl). But there was little interest in this role for potassium until the 1980s, during which 19 controlled trials were reported, most of double blind crossover design. A meta-analysis of these shows that oral KCl usually lowers systolic and diastolic blood pressure, and does so more in hypertensive than normotensive people. There are, however, two limitations to the applicability of these trials to dietary management of blood pressure. The first is that the potassium supplements have usually been at a dose of 50 to 100 mmol/day and there are very few foods that are rich enough in potassium to provide this intake by incorporating them in a diet. Secondly, if patients have managed to bring their sodium intake down below to around 70 mmol/day, the hypotensive effect of extra potassium may be trivial.

Body Weight

In a follow-up study of over 5,000 people born in Britain in one week of March 1946, examinations at the age of 36 found that blood pressures were progressively higher above a body mass index (kg weight ÷ [height in metres]^2) of 25, i.e. in those classifiable as overweight. This association of higher blood pressure in fatter people is a general experience, reported in many cross-sectional and prospective studies. There is a tendency for falsely high readings of blood pressure by indirect measurement using the usual cuff, but in Framingham the correlation between blood pressure and relative weight was still seen when the sphygmomanometer cuff was placed around the forearm and sounds heard over the radial artery. Typically a 3 mm Hg higher systolic pressure may be expected for every 10 kg increase in body weight. In a large Swedish study of 60-year-old men, a quarter of the fattest fifth (quintile) were taking antihypertensive drugs compared with only 4 per cent of the thinnest fifth.

People who don't eat enough food energy and lose body weight usually have a fall of blood pressure, even people of normal weight and blood pressure. If hypertensive overweight people reduce their weight they show falls of blood pressure such as 10 mm systolic/5 mm diastolic for 5 kg weight loss. Less food normally means less salt eaten, but blood pressure falls with weight reduction even if sodium intake is maintained. Weight loss is accompanied by reductions in plasma renin activity and aldosterone levels, irrespective of sodium intake.

In a randomized placebo-controlled trial of first-line treatment of mild hypertension in overweight patients, the weight reduction group (mean loss 7.4 kg) had a 13 mm Hg fall of systolic blood pressure while those treated with metoprolol (a beta adrenergic blocker) had a 10 mm Hg fall. Plasma lipids improved in the weight reduction group but changed adversely in those on drug therapy.[43]

Alcohol

Apart from an observation on soldiers in France in 1915 which seems to have been ignored, the association of alcohol consumption with higher blood pressure started to be noted in the late 1960s. In cross-sectional data of over 80,000 health examinations in California,[44] this association was significant, it appeared independent, and there was a threshold: blood pressure did not increase until three drinks per day. This phenomenon has been confirmed in a number of large epidemiological studies. The curve may be J-shaped, i.e. lower blood pressure at one or two drinks per day than in teetotallers. The association in women was not clear in one study, probably because this was a population sample, with few heavy-drinking women.

Clinical and experimental investigations have shown that in alcoholics admitted to hospital for detoxification blood pressure is usually raised on admission and usually falls to normal within a week. In those who continue to abstain at follow-up, blood pressure remains normal but it goes up again in those who relapse. Puddey et al. in Perth (Australia) have demonstrated by the use of low alcohol beer, a direct effect of alcohol consumption on normotensive moderate drinkers[45] and on hypertensive heavier drinkers.[46]

The effect of alcohol on blood pressure is predominantly due to alcohol consumed in the few days immediately preceding the blood pressure measurement. The mechanism for the effect of alcohol is not yet established. Possibilities include increased cortisol secretion and increased red cell volume.

Polyunsaturated Fat

Workers in Finland in 1983 reported a randomized dietary crossover trial in the community in North Karelia. In the group who took a 23 per cent fat (energy) diet and increased proportion of polyunsaturated fat (omega-6) blood pressure fell.[47] There were more changes in the diet than simply the fatty acids (e.g. lower dietary cholesterol, more vegetables). Beilin's group in Perth found in a well-controlled trial in hospital staff that blood pressure was lower on a lacto-ovo-vegetarian diet than on an omnivorous diet.[48] Sodium intakes were held the same. Type of fat was one of the nutritional differences between the diets. The group went on to test the effect of changing only the ratio of polyunsaturated to saturated fatty acids. Blood pressure was not lower on the higher polyunsaturated (omega-6) fatty acid diet.

From 1981 there have been 21 trials with long chain omega-3 polyunsaturated fatty acids in the form of cod liver oil (2), Max EPA (11), fatty fish (4) or different preparations of fish oil (3) on blood pressure. In most of the experiments with fish oil, blood pressure fell, diastolic or systolic or both, provided the dose of omega-3 fatty acids, eicosapentaenoic (20:5) plus docosahexaenoic (22:6) was above 3 g/day. In several experiments capsules of a vegetable oil were used as a control, usually olive oil, although an omega-6 polyunsaturated oil was used in two experiments. With fish, e.g. 100 g/day of mackerel, there was no effect except with 280 g/day of canned mackerel.

Thus any effect of omega-6 polyunsaturated fatty acids proved elusive and an effect of the marine omega-3 polyunsaturates is only seen with exceptionally large intakes of fatty fish or with concentrated fish oil preparations.

Calcium

Calcium inside cells has an important effect on membrane stability and smooth muscle tone. Calcium and sodium interact at many levels. For example, calcium is exchanged for sodium in one of the systems that adjust ion concentrations in the cell. When sodium intake is high, more calcium is lost in the urine; thiazide diuretics increase urinary sodium excretion but decrease calcium loss. Intracellular calcium is a major determinant of arteriolar smooth muscle tone and hence blood pressure; this is the basis for the action of calcium channel blocking drugs like nifedipine.

Addison[49] first reported that increased calcium intake could lower blood pressure in patients with essential hypertension in 1924. This observation was largely ignored. McCarron from 1982[50,51] presented a well-reasoned hypothesis that dietary calcium may protect against hypertension. Evidence included reports of less hypertension in hard water areas and an apparent lower calcium intake in asymptomatic people with hypertension in the large US nutrition and health examination survey (NHANES) (carried out in the early 1970s). McCarron reported a single case of hypertension, on very low calcium intake, whose blood pressure fell promptly when advised to increase dairy food consumption. His analysis of NHANES data was criticized by senior scientists associated with the survey and some reported findings are hard to reconcile with the hypothesis, for example a positive relation of serum (total) calcium to blood pressure.

By 1990 a review of 25 observational epidemiological studies shows some supporting McCarron's hypothesis, some not and considerable inconsistency. But in the only purely prospective study of dietary factors, including calcium, in relation to blood pressure, the Nurses' Health Study,[52] the relative risk of (self-reported) hypertension for a calcium intake at or above the recommended daily allowance (RDA) (800 mg/d) was 0.78 compared with an intake of less than 400 mg/d. During the 1980s a number of intervention trials were done with oral calcium supplements. Twenty-one trials have been reported (some in two sections) in hypertensives and/or normotensives. Three meta-analyses, each using somewhat different selection criteria and way of presentation, show a very small mean reducing effect of added calcium on systolic blood pressure, standing rather than supine. In an additional recent trial, a few hypertensive patients responded to calcium carbonate (as against placebo) but after three months off extra calcium, on re-challenge the response did not occur the second time.

Combined nutritional treatment is thus an important section of the range of treatments available now for high blood pressure: weight reduction for anyone at all overweight, reduction of alcohol to only one or two drinks a day and reduction of salt to 70 mmol or less sodium per day. (This can be monitored by 24-hour urine collection). Combined nutritional therapy, to which can be added regular exercise and measures to help relaxation, is the best treatment for someone with questionable high blood pressure; it may be the only treatment needed for mild hypertension and, for more severe hypertension, it enables the dose of drugs to be lower, resulting in fewer side-effects. Older people may be more responsive to salt reduction and they are particularly susceptible to side-effects of drugs. As the US Department of Health and Human Sciences report puts it: 'Nonpharmacologic interventions for management of both hypertension and high blood cholesterol are recognised as the essential first step of therapy'.[53]

NOTES

1 Aschoff, L. (1906) *Verhandelung Deutsche Gesellschaft für Pathologie* 10, 166, quoted by Schönheimer, R. (1928) 'Zur Chemie der gesunden und der atherosklerotischen Aorta', *Zeitschrift für Physiologische Chemie* 177, 143–57.
2 Keys, A., Kimura, N., Kusukawa, A., Bronte-Stewart, B., Larsen, N. and Keys, M. H. (1958) 'Lessons from serum cholesterol studies in Japan, Hawaii and Los Angeles', *Annals of Internal Medicine* 48, 83–94.
3 Kannel, W. B., Castelli, W. P., Gordon, T. and McNamara, P. M. (1971) 'Serum cholesterol, lipoproteins and the risk of coronary heart disease. The Framingham Study', *Annals of Internal Medicine* 74, 1–12.
4 Keys, A. (1952) 'The cholesterol problem', *Voeding* 13, 539–55.
5 Mellinkoff, S. M., Marchella, T. A. and Reinhold, J. G. (1950) 'The effect of a fat-free diet in causing low serum cholesterol', *American Journal of Medical Science* 220, 203–7.
6 Kempner, W. (1946) 'Some effects of rice diet treatment of kidney disease and hypertension', *Bulletin of the New York Academy of Medicine* 22, 358–70.
7 Bronte-Stewart, B., Keys, A., Brock, J. F., Moodie, A. D., Keys, M. H. and Antonis, A. (1955) 'Serum cholesterol, diet and coronary heart-disease: an inter-racial survey in the Cape Peninsula', *Lancet* 269, 1103–8.
8 Bronte-Stewart, B., Antonis, A., Fales, L. and Brock, J. F. (1956) 'Effects of feeding different fats on serum-cholesterol levels', *Lancet* 1, 521–7.
9 Keys, A. (1970) (ed.) 'Coronary heart disease in seven countries', *Circulation*, Supplement 1 to vols 41 and 42, 211 pp.
10 Mensink, R. P. and Katan, M. B. (1989) 'Effect of a diet enriched with monounsaturated or polyunsaturated fatty acids on levels of low-density and high-density lipoprotein cholesterol in healthy men and women', *New England Journal of Medicine* 321, 436–41.
11 Mensink, R. P. and Katan, M. B. (1990) 'Effect of dietary trans-fatty acids on high-level and low-density lipoprotein cholesterol levels in healthy subjects', *New England Journal of Medicine* 323, 439–45.
12 Truswell, A. S. (1990) 'Malnutrition and carbohydrate and lipid metabolism', in R. T. M. Suskind and L. L. Suskind (eds) *The Malnourished Child*, Vevey, Nestlé/New York, Raven Press, pp. 95–115.
13 Report of the Advisory Panel of the Committee on Medical Aspects of Food Policy (Nutrition), Department of Health and Social Security (1974) Diet and Coronary Heart Disease. Report on Health and Social Subjects 7, London, HMSO.
14 Truswell, A. S. (1987) 'Sugar and health: a review', *Food Technology in Australia*, 39, 134–40.

15 Report of the Panel on Dietary Sugars, Committee on Medical Aspects of Food Policy, Department of Health (1989) Dietary Sugars and Human Disease. Report on Health and Social Subjects 37, London, HMSO.
16 Trowell, H. (1972) 'Ischaemic heart disease and dietary fiber', *American Journal of Clinical Nutrition* 25, 926–32.
17 Truswell, A. S. and Beynen, A. C. (1992) 'Dietary fibre and plasma lipids: potential for prevention and treatment of hyperlipidaemias', in T. F. Schweizer and C. A. Edwards (eds) *Dietary Fibre – A Component of Food. Nutritional function in health and disease*, London, Berlin, Heidelberg, Springer-Verlag, pp. 295–332.
18 Report of a Joint Working Party of the Royal College of Physicians of London and the British Cardiac Society (1976) 'Prevention of coronary heart disease', *Journal of the Royal College of Physicians* 10, 213–75.
19 Kannel, W. B., Le Bauer, E. J., Dawber, T. R. and McNamara, P. M. (1967) 'Relation of body weight to development of coronary heart disease', *Circulation* 35, 734–44.
20 Klatsky, A. L., Friedman, G. D. and Siegelaub, A. B. (1974) 'Alcohol consumption before myocardial infarction. Results from the Kaiser-Permanente epidemiologic study of myocardial infarction', *Annals of Internal Medicine* 81, 294–301.
21 Jick, H., Miettinen, O. S., Neff, R. K., Shapiro, S., Heinonen, O. P. and Slone, D. (1973) 'Coffee and myocardial infarction', *New England Journal of Medicine* 289, 63–7.
22 Førde, O. H., Knutsen, S. F., Arnesen, E. and Thelle, D. S. (1985) 'The Tromsø heart study: coffee consumption and serum lipid concentrations in men with hypercholesterolaemia: a randomised intervention study', *British Medical Journal* 290, 893–5.
23 Zock, P. L., Katan, M. B., Merkus, M. P., van Dusseldorp, M. and Harryvan, J. L. (1990) 'Effect of a lipid-rich fraction from boiled coffee on serum cholesterol', *Lancet* 335, 1235–7.
24 La Croix, A. Z., Mead, L. A., Liang, K.-L., Thomas, C. B. and Pearson, T. A. (1986) 'Coffee consumption and the incidence of coronary heart disease', *New England Journal of Medicine* 315, 977–82.
25 Editorial (1969) 'The water story', *Lancet* 1, 1012–13.
26 Pocock, S. J., Shaper, A. G., Cook, D. G., Packham, R. F., Lacey, R. F., Powell, P. and Russell, P. F. (1980) 'British Regional Heart Study: geographical variations in cardiovascular mortality, and the role of water quality', *British Medical Journal* 1, 1243–9.
27 Wood, D. A., Riemersma, R. A., Butler, S., Thompson, M., MacIntyre, C., Elton, R. A. and Oliver, M. F. (1987) 'Linoleic and eicosapentaenoic acids in adipose tissue and platelets and risk of coronary heart disease', *Lancet* 1, 177–82.
28 Osler, W. and McCrae, T. (1913) *The Principles and Practice of Medicine* 8th edn, New York and London, D. Appleton and Co., pp. 426–39.
29 Graham, G. (1930) 'Diseases of metabolism', in F. W. Price (ed.) *A Textbook of the Practice of Medicine* 3rd edn, London, Oxford University Press, pp. 412–20.
30 Abrahams, M. and Widdowson, E. M. (1940) *Modern Dietary Treatment* 2nd edn, London, Baillière, Tindall and Cox.

31 Cahill, G. F. (1975) 'Diabetes mellitus', in P. B. Beeson and W. McDermott (eds) *Textbook of Medicine* 14th edn, Philadelphia, London and Toronto, W. B. Saunders, pp. 1599–1619.

32 Joslin, E. P. (1928) *The Treatment of Diabetes Mellitus* 4th edn, Philadelphia, Lea and Febiger.

33 Himsworth, H. P. (1935–6) 'The influence of diet on the sugar tolerance of healthy men and its reference to certain extrinsic factors', *Clinical Science* 2, 67–94.

34 Trowell, H. (1974) 'Diabetes mellitus death rates in England and Wales 1920–70 and food supplies', *Lancet* 2, 998–1002.

35 Jenkins, D. J. A., Wolever, T. M. S., Hockaday, T. D. R., Leeds, A. R., Howart, R., Bacon, S., Apling, E. C. and Dilawari, J. (1977) 'Treatment of diabetes with guar gum', *Lancet* 2, 779–80.

36 Brand, J. C., Colagiuri, S., Crossman, S., Allen, A., Roberts, D. C. K. and Truswell, A. S. (1991) 'Low-glycaemic index foods improve long-term glycaemic control in NIDDM', *Diabetes Care* 14, 95–101.

37 Ambard, L. and Beaujard, E. (1904) 'Causes de l'hypertension artérielle', *Archives Générales de Médecine* 1, 520.

38 Allen, F. M. (1922) 'Treatment of arterial hypertension', *Medical Clinics of North America* 6, 475–81.

39 Dole, V. P., Dahl, L. K., Cotzias, G. C., Dziewiatkowski, D. D. and Harris, C. (1951) 'Dietary treatment of hypertension. II. Sodium depletion as related to the therapeutic effect', *Journal of Clinical Investigation* 30, 584–95.

40 Addison, W. L. T. (1928) 'The use of sodium chloride, potassium chloride, sodium bromide and potassium bromide in cases of arterial hypertension which are amenable to potassium chloride', *Canadian Medical Association Journal* 18, 281–5.

41 Priddle, W. W. (1931) 'Observations on the management of hypertension', *Canadian Medical Association Journal* 25, 5–8.

42 McQuarrie, I., Thompson, W. H. and Anderson, J. A. (1936) 'Effects of excessive ingestion of sodium and potassium salts on carbohydrate metabolism and blood pressure in diabetic children', *Journal of Nutrition* 11, 77–101.

43 MacMahon, S. W., Macdonald, G. J., Bernstein, L., Andrews, G. and Blackett, R. B. (1985) 'Comparison of weight reduction with metoprolol in treatment of hypertension in young overweight patients', *Lancet* 1, 1233–6.

44 Klatsky, A. L., Friedman, G. D., Siegelaub, A. B. and Gérard, M. J. (1977) 'Alcohol consumption and blood pressure. Kaiser-Permanente multiphasic health examination data', *New England Journal of Medicine* 296, 1194–1200.

45 Puddey, I. B., Beilin, L. J., Vandongen, R., Rouse, I. L. and Rogers, P. (1985) 'Evidence for a direct effect of alcohol consumption on blood pressure in normotensive men. A randomized controlled trial', *Hypertension* 7, 707–13.

46 Puddey, I. B., Beilin, L. J. and Vandongen, R. (1987) 'Regular alcohol use raises blood pressure in treated hypertensive subjects', *Lancet* 1, 647–51.

47 Puska, P., Iacono, J. M., Nissinen, A., Korhonen, J. H., Vartiainen, E., Pietinen, P., Dougherty, R., Leino, U., Mutanen, M., Moisio, S. and Huttunen, J. (1983) 'Controlled, randomised trial of the effect of dietary fat on blood pressure', *Lancet* 1, 1–5.

48 Rouse, I. L., Beilin, L. J., Armstrong, B. K. and Vandongen, R. (1983) Blood

pressure-lowering effect of a vegetarian diet: controlled trial in normotensive subjects', *Lancet* 1, 5–10.

49 Addison, W. L. T. (1924) 'The use of calcium chloride in arterial hypertension', *Canadian Medical Association Journal* 14, 1059–61.

50 McCarron, D. A., Morris, C. D. and Cole, C. (1982) 'Dietary calcium in human hypertension', *Science* 217, 267–9.

51 McCarron, D. A. (1983) 'Calcium and magnesium nutrition in human hypertension', *Annals of Internal Medicine* 98 (2), 800–5.

52 Witteman, J. C. M., Willett, W. C., Stampfer, M. J., Colditz, G. A., Sacks, F. M., Speizer, F. E., Rosner, B. and Hennekens, C. H. (1989) 'A prospective study of nutritional factors and hypertension among US women', *Circulation* 80, 1320–7.

53 National High Blood Pressure Education Program (NHBPEP) and National Cholesterol Education Program (NCEP): Working Group Report on Management of Patients with Hypertension and High Blood Cholesterol (1990) NIH Publication No. 90-2361, US Department of Health and Human Services.

Readers who require the full set of 244 references for this chapter are invited to contact the author.

4

Diseases of Diet in Affluent Societies

John Garrow

The most important causes of death among adults in affluent countries, such as the UK, are cardiovascular diseases (coronary thrombosis, high blood pressure, stroke and congestive heart failure) and cancer, which account for 21 per cent and 26 per cent respectively of years of life lost up to age 65 years.[1] Important causes of disability are respiratory and musculo-skeletal diseases, and non-insulin-dependent diabetes mellitus (NIDDM). These diseases are all essentially degenerative diseases: they occur as organs and tissues wear out or cease to obey the normal rules of cell replication. They are also diseases in which the aetiology is linked with diet. Other chapters deal with the nutritional and economic aspects of food, or the absence of food: this chapter is concerned with the paradox that, in affluent countries such as the UK, where choice of food for the majority of the population is not constrained by availability or economic factors, so many important diseases are largely attributable to diet. Part of the explanation is that in Third World countries, undernutrition and infectious diseases account for many deaths in young people, whereas these causes of mortality are almost eliminated in affluent countries. However, even when our mortality rates are standardized for age, the commonest causes of death are the degenerative and malignant diseases: the diseases of diet in affluent countries are also typically the diseases of old age.

Why should the rich person seeking pleasure (and presumably also longevity) choose a diet which leads to premature aging of the tissues? Two popular explanations can be dismissed at once, since they seem to be based on a certain view of social justice, but do not fit the nutritional facts. It may be true that the richest individuals use (or abuse) their wealth to obtain excessive quantities of the richest food and drink, which do them no good, but this theory cannot explain why the diseases of diet in affluent societies fall most heavily on its least affluent members. The second theory contains at least an element of the truth: that humans evolved to eat a certain type

Table 4.1 The effect of affluence on food supply

	Peasant poverty	*Urban affluence*
Quantity of food	Limited Intermittent	Unlimited* Constant
Transport and storage	Poor and unsatisfactory (e.g. by salting)	Excellent (by packaging, canning freezing, use of additives)
Variety	Limited	Unlimited*
Contamination	Bacteria, insects parasites	Antibiotics pesticides, additives

*Aspects of food supply most closely associated with diseases.

of diet which was full of natural goodness, but in affluent countries all but the very rich are forced to eat food from which most of the goodness has been processed out. This theory casts the food industry as villains who wilfully foist pseudo-food on the masses, thereby committing genocide. My experience of people in the food industry suggests that they have a policy similar to that of other industrialists: killing the customer is to be avoided if possible for commercial, as well as humanitarian, reasons.

So, it is the diet of the average person in affluent countries rather than that of its rich members which leads to degenerative diseases. I believe that the key to the problem lies in the change in social organization which is inevitably associated with increasing affluence in the community. Waterlow[2] has made an interesting comparison of the cost of food in Rome in 302 AD with the cost of food in London in 1988 AD. The inhabitant of ancient Rome needed to spend about one tenth of an average daily wage to buy enough flour to satisfy normal energy requirements (say 10 MJ), whereas the same amount of flour would cost the modern Londoner only one five-hundredth of an average daily wage. To buy pork, mutton, chicken, cheese, oil or wine, the ancient Roman would have to spend more than ten times the cost of an equal weight of flour, while in modern times these foods cost about four times the price of flour. Thus affluence enables ordinary people to buy more food, with greater variety. Table 4.1 contrasts the features of the food supply in a poor country, where individuals or families hunt, grow or gather food for their own consumption – the 'peasant poverty' scenario – with that in an affluent country where most people live in conurbations and buy their food, which has been produced by unknown people who live far away.

Table 4.1 shows that in almost all respects the food supply for the city-dweller is far better than that for the peasant: abundant varied food available at any time as against an uncertain supply of monotonous food which is difficult to store. Some people maintain that the risk of contamination of food with antibiotics administered to animals, with pesticides sprayed on crops, or with additives which are designed to improve the appearance, taste or keeping qualities of food, is a serious cause for concern. I am not convinced that this is a significant risk, given the food safety regulations which are designed to prevent such contamination reaching dangerous levels; in any case, the threat is probably far less than that from the type of contamination present in unprocessed food. Unexpectedly, it seems that the diseases of diet in affluent countries are most strongly related to the two features of the food supply which appear most obviously beneficial: the unlimited supply of food in virtually unlimited variety.

Regulation of *ad libitum* Food Intake

The classical approach to studying mechanisms which effect physiological regulation in the body is to investigate the system by experimental manipulation in a lower animal, such as the laboratory rat. As recently as 1973, a major textbook of human nutrition[3] described in detail the areas of the hypothalamus which control the eating behaviour of a rat fed on laboratory chow. Lesions in different areas of the hypothalamus would cause the rat to regulate food intake to maintain a higher, or lower, body weight. However, it was admitted that it was not certain if these neural pathways really controlled energy intake in humans, nor was it clear what mechanism was responsible for the signal to stop eating. Lane-Petter[4] asked the pertinent question: Do laboratory animals like eating? A rat is said to be satiated when it shows no inclination to eat laboratory chow, which human subjects would have been unwilling to eat anyway. If the 'satiated' rat is offered more palatable food, such as chocolate, it will again eat.

In the 1970s and 1980s considerable advances have been made in our understanding of the factors which control energy intake in man when offered a varied, palatable diet. When we eat, the food is absorbed from the gut and there are many potential signals which might cause satiety: it has been suggested that the important messengers might be products of the digestion of food (such as glucose) entering the bloodstream, or nerve signals arising from the gut as food is absorbed, or hormones released from the gut wall in response to the presence of food in the gut lumen. The problem with all these suggestions is that they do not explain how the last mouthful of a meal is determined: the signals listed above require that food should already be in the intestine, if not actually absorbed, before the signal can be generated, but while this is happening there is time for many more mouthfuls to be ingested before the meal is terminated.

A solution to this problem is offered in a study by Booth et al.[5] Normal volunteers were given meals consisting of a lemon-flavoured drink, sandwiches, and a dessert of yoghurt. The lemon-flavoured drink had on some days 65 g starch, and on other days 5 g starch, but these were indistinguishable by taste or appearance. The dessert yoghurt was in two flavours, of which one was given on the days when there was a large starch preload, and the other when there was a small starch preload. After some days the volunteers reliably ate less sandwiches and yoghurt after the high than after the low preload. This phase of the experiment showed that the volunteers were able to respond to a covert alteration in the starch preload by altering voluntary food intake thereafter.

In the second phase of the experiment the volunteers were given a 35 g starch preload at all meals, but it was observed that (for a few days) they ate less on the days when they were served the yoghurt flavour previously associated with the high preload than when they were served the yoghurt previously associated with the low preload. This result showed that satiety in these circumstances is to some extent *conditioned*: the subjects felt full after less food because the yoghurt flavour was associated with an experience of earlier satiety in the previous phase of the experiment.

Another insight into the nature of satiety was provided by Rolls et al.[6] Normal volunteers were offered a four-course meal consisting of sausages, then bread and butter, then a chocolate dessert, and finally bananas, and the weight of food consumed at each course, and its energy value, was recorded. On other occasions the volunteers were offered similar food as four courses, but each course consisted of the same food item: thus there would be a meal of sausage, followed by sausage, followed by sausage, and then sausage, and so on for each of the other items on the menu. The total weight of food was 44 per cent greater, and energy intake was 60 per cent greater, when the meal had four different types of food than when it had only one. This is a formal demonstration of a principle which underlies gastronomy: that an appetising meal should provide variety and contrasts in taste, colour and texture. It is a common experience that, having partaken of a banquet which provided much more nourishment than we need, we may believe ourselves to be incapable of eating any more. However, if a particularly attractive item is produced – perhaps the first strawberries of the season – we find the ability to eat is miraculously restored.

These findings show that novelty and variety in food makes it more difficult to regulate intake by physiological mechanisms. If, like the laboratory rat, we were fed chow of constant composition, we would no doubt regulate our food intake accurately according to our requirements. We would do this because at each meal we would acquire experience about the quantity of food which fulfilled our needs, and having ingested that amount we would feel satiated by the conditioning effect demonstrated by Booth et al. However, this mechanism works only for meals of which we have had previous experience. If each meal is novel, we have no experience of that meal with which conditioning of satiety can occur. If our cuisine is varied as well as novel the task of regulation is made still more difficult, because satiety is 'sensory specific': we may be satiated to sausages but not yet satiated to bananas. The application of this theory to diet in affluent countries is obvious: food technologists are constantly inventing new flavours and textures which may not exist in any natural food, with the laudable intention of stimulating both our appetites and their sales. It is not surprising that the physiological mechanism which evolved to regulate intake of the monotonous diet of our ancestors is no match for such sophistication.

Biological Advantages of Sensory-specific Satiety and of Fat Storage

Sensory-specific satiety is not a design error on the part of God. It must have urged our ancestors to eat a variety of foods and not just to eat the large animal which they had recently killed, or the stem of bananas which had recently become ripe. In this way the quality of the diet is improved, because the more different foods there are in a diet, the less likely it is that there will be an overall deficiency of specific nutrients such as vitamins or essential amino acids. It is therefore a great advantage to the poor peasant whose food supply is limited, monotonous and intermittent, and for whom the main nutritional danger is undernutrition.

The evolutionary success of mammalian species is due partly to their ability to regulate their internal body temperature, and thus operate in low ambient temperature which would immobilize poikilothermic animals, and partly to the ability to suckle their young and provide optimum nutrition at a very vulnerable stage of the life cycle. The regulation of body temperature in a cold environment, and the production of breast milk, are both processes requiring energy. Mammals have energy stores, mainly in the form of a layer of subcutaneous fat, which enables them to perform these essential functions even in conditions in which the food supply is temporarily inadequate. It follows that they must also have the ability to replenish these stores at times when the food supply is more than enough to satisfy current requirements.

Overeating, Overweight, Obesity and Excess Mortality

The ample and varied food supply in affluent countries tends to promote a greater food intake than would have been the case on a limited monotonous diet. However, it is not easy to define 'overeating' in a meal-eating mammal such as man. Energy intake is intermittent during the day, but energy expenditure is continuous. An individual who maintains weight over a long period is constantly oscillating between periods of excess energy intake (immediately after a meal) and excess energy output (immediately before the next meal). Within reasonable limits, it is desirable that there should be energy stored as fat for the reasons given above, and as a reserve in times of famine. At any moment the energy economy of the body is controlled in such a way that energy demands are met, and dietary energy intake is apportioned to immediate use, or to storage, or (in children) to growth. A central role in the management of fuel use in the body is played by the hormone insulin.

Overweight is defined operationally by the experience of insurance companies. Since the beginning of the twentieth century, actuaries have noted that people who were above a given weight for height tended to die young, and hence were unprofitable to insure. Doctors examining candidates for life insurance were given guidelines about the range of 'desirable' weight for a given height. The excess mortality among men who were overweight was usually due to heart disease. Men who had been charged excess premiums because they were overweight, but who then reduced to desirable weight, subsequently had normal life expectancy. It seemed reasonable on this evidence to conclude that obesity somehow caused heart disease. It was also assumed that a fat person was fat because, as Dr Samuel Johnson said with characteristic bluntness, 'he has eaten more than he should have done.'[7]

Some further investigations of the relationship between overeating, overweight, obesity and heart disease greatly complicated the matter. First, it was shown that overweight was not necessarily equivalent to obesity: Behnke et al.[8] showed that some national-ranking football players, who had been refused for service in the US armed forces because they were overweight, were not fat, but heavily muscled. Next, it was reported that obese high school girls actually had a *lower* energy intake than lean controls, so it was concluded that their obesity must be due to a low level of physical activity.[9] Finally, a large investigation into causes of heart disease among men in seven different countries seemed to show that the important risk factors were age, cigarette smoking, blood pressure and serum cholesterol concentration: if these factors were known, the addition of any measure of adiposity did not contribute to the equations for predicting which men would have a heart attack.[10] It was therefore concluded that obesity was not in itself a risk factor; it just happened that the risk factors named above often occurred in obese people.

However, the picture has now become clearer again, and it emerges that the intuitive conclusions of the early 1940s were near to the truth. While it is true that certain classes of people, such as professional athletes, may be overweight due to an excess of muscle, in the great majority of people who are overweight the excess tissue is 75 per cent fat and 25 per cent fat-free mass.[11] In a series of 104 women and 24 men, fatness explained more than 90 per cent of variation in weight for a given height. While it is true that obese people often *report* a lower food intake than lean controls, this is not compatible with measurement of energy expenditure. Several studies using different methods for estimating daily energy expenditure in obese and lean subjects have consistently shown that the obese group has a significantly *higher* energy output, regardless of the level of physical activity, so thermodynamic considerations require that they must also have a higher energy intake in order to maintain body weight.[12] Thus we can now say with some confidence that overweight (except in some classes of athletes) is equivalent to obesity, and that obesity is, in general, due to overeating.

The relationship of obesity to disease, and particularly heart disease, is quite complex. The multiple regression analysis of Keys et al.[10] found that age, cigarette smoking, blood pressure and serum cholesterol concentration were the risk factors for heart disease. The increasing risk with age and cigarette smoking is not in doubt. However, high blood pressure and serum cholesterol (particularly the increased low-density fraction, and decreased protective high-density fraction) are highly correlated with obesity.[13] If obesity increases the risk of heart disease mainly by increasing blood pressure and altering unfavourable the distribution of cholesterol fractions, then an analysis which has taken the latter two factors into account will see little effect remaining for obesity *per se*. In fact obesity does contribute to heart disease directly, even when allowance is made for age, blood pressure, smoking, cholesterol and ventricular hypertrophy, but it takes many years for this independent effect to become detectable.[14] The pathways by which obesity, in association with other lifestyle factors, contributes to heart disease are indicated in figure 4.1.

How Obesity Causes Disease

Recent work on animal models of obesity has shown that the primary metabolic defect is a reduced sensitivity to insulin, from which all the other metabolic characteristics associated with obesity follow.[15] The classic study of Sims and colleagues[16] in Vermont showed that if experimental obesity is produced by prolonged overfeeding of normal men, with no family history of diabetes, a similar syndrome of insulin insensitivity is produced, which reverts to normal with weight loss. Susceptibility to arterial disease increases in parallel with increasing glucose intolerance,[17] so this is one route by which obesity predisposes to cardiovascular disease. Glucose intolerance, or serum insulin concentration, is highly correlated with hypertension,[18] so this is another route. Regardless of insulin insensitivity, obesity is

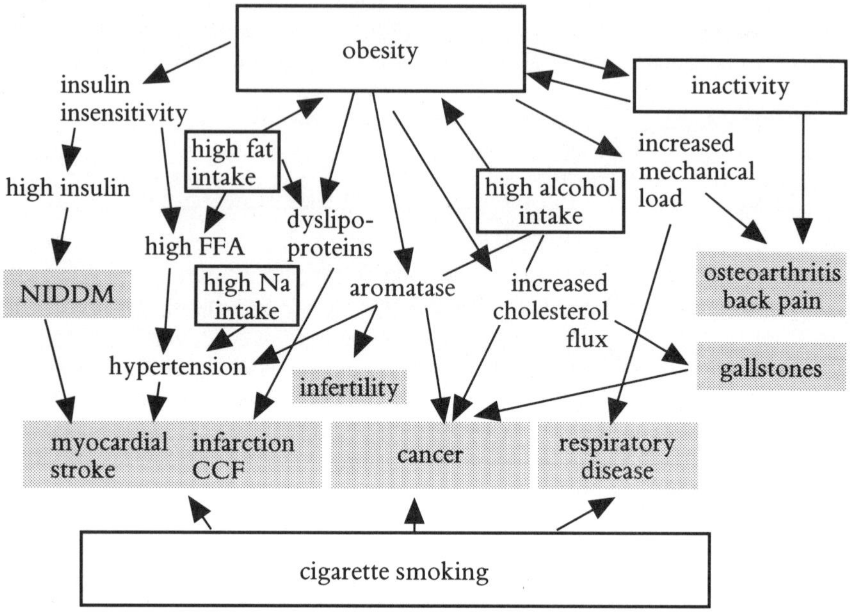

Figure 4.1 Pathways by which obesity contributes to heart disease. Shaded boxes indicate diet-related diseases, and white boxes indicate changeable aspects of lifestyle which increase the risk of these diseases. Arrows indicate causative pathways, and items not in boxes are intermediate mechanisms by which the lifestyle factors affect the risk of disease. Factors which are important in determining disease risk, but which cannot be altered by the individual (such as age and genetic make-up) are not shown. (FFA = free fatty acids, NIDDM = non-insulin-dependent diabetes mellitus, CCF = chronic congestive heart failure.)

associated with an unfavourable plasma lipoprotein pattern, with high LDL-cholesterol and triglycerides and low HDL-cholesterol,[19,13] so this is a third route linking obesity with cardiovascular disease.

Another route by which obesity causes disease arises because adipose tissue contains the enzyme system aromatase, which converts androgens into oestrogens.[12] The resulting hormonal imbalance contributes to infertility and polycystic ovarian syndrome which are common complications of obesity, and also probably explains the increased prevalence of sex-hormone-sensitive cancers in obese people.[20] Adipose tissue is also an important reservoir of cholesterol, so obese people have a greatly increased cholesterol flux and supersaturated bile,[21] which makes them liable to form gallstones, have abnormal liver function[22] and gallbladder cancer.

Finally, the increased body weight associated with obesity contributes to the reduced exercise tolerance and respiratory problems of obese people, and the increased liability to musculoskeletal diseases and osteoarthritis of weight-bearing joints.[12,23]

Other Lifestyle Factors which Contribute to Disease in Affluent Countries

In figure 4.1, there are other factors which work together with obesity to increase the risk of disease. These are inactivity, and a high intake of alcohol, saturated fat and salt. It is not difficult to see an association between these risks and the social organization of affluent countries.

The poor peasant is forced to adopt a physically active lifestyle every day in order to secure his or her food supply, whereas the affluent city worker has only to push a trolley round the supermarket to collect all the food needed for a week. Alcohol, saturated fat and salt are all dietary components which tend to be associated with improved keeping quality of foodstuffs: alcohol in high concentration is an antiseptic, and saturated fat has less tendency than unsaturated fat to become rancid. Salt, or sugar in high concentration, stops spoiling of food by bacterial growth by limiting the free water available to contaminating organisms. Meats and fish can be preserved by salting, and fruit by making into a jam with a high concentration of sugar. Chocolate consists of a mixture of cocoa fat and sugar with very little water, and has good keeping qualities. Thus it happens that the components of food which assist storage tend to be associated with diet-related diseases, but it is essential that food should keep well if it is to be transported to the affluent city-dweller from the distant places where it is produced. Conversely, the foods which tend to be protective against diseases, such as fresh fruit and vegetables, are notoriously difficult to store and transport without expensive protection such as freezing.

Recent Changes in Dietary Risk Factors and in Disease Prevalence

One of the most difficult challenges to those who offer advice about healthy nutrition is to demonstrate the validity of their advice, especially when it concerns avoiding the diseases of affluent countries, which are essentially degenerative diseases. These diseases take a long time to develop, so it is necessary to manipulate risk factors for a long time before it is reasonable to expect to see benefit. Sceptics will want to see positive results in a

Table 4.2 Prevalence (%) of obesity (Quetelet's Index > 30 kg/m^2) in a representative sample of men and women in the United Kingdom in 1980 and 1987

	Men		*Women*	
Age (years)	*1980*	*1987*	*1980*	*1987*
16–24	2.5	3.0	3.5	6.0
25–34	4.5	6.0	4.5	11.0
35–49	8.0	11.0	9.9	10.0
50–64	7.7	9.0	14.3	18.0

Data of Rosenbaum et al.[28] and of Gregory et al.[29]

population in which the advice has been followed before following the advice themselves, but where can a population of non-sceptics be found to provide this evidence? Huge sums of money have been spent on multiple risk factor intervention trials, which have demonstrated moderate benefits and which have been variously interpreted. Some say they show that the risk factors have only a weak effect, or that the control group also followed similar advice, or that the intervention group complied imperfectly.

Concerning obesity, there is rather clear evidence of benefit with weight loss. In the Vermont experiment, the insulin insensitivity produced by experimental obesity returned to normal with weight loss,[16] and the obese diabetic shows improved diabetic control and improved blood lipids with weight loss.[24] Spontaneous weight change in whole populations is highly significantly associated with change in risk factors such as blood pressure, cholesterol, triglycerides, fasting and post-prandial glucose, uric acid and forced vital capacity,[25,26] and a randomized controlled trial of weight reduction versus propanolol in young overweight hypertensive adults showed better results with weight reduction than with the drug.[27]

Unfortunately the prevalence of obesity (defined as $W/H^2 > 30$) in the UK is increasing at an alarming rate. Table 4.2 shows the prevalence among men and women in 1980 and in 1987. Overall the prevalence has increased from 6 per cent and 8 per cent in 1980 to 8 per cent and 12 per cent in 1987 in men and women respectively.

How to Get the Benefits of Affluence without the Dietary Diseases

Most of the differences between the diet of poor and affluent communities are to the advantage of the affluent, so it would be folly to suggest that we should revert to the monotonous, uncertain and unsafe food supply of the poor peasant. The main dangers of the affluent diet are overconsumption of energy and underconsumption of some of the more perishable types of food, such as fresh fruit and vegetables. Other aspects which require attention are an inadequate intake of cereal fibre, which may predispose to constipation and other forms of bowel disease, and overconsumption of both sucrose, which predisposes to dental caries, and alcohol, which is a liver poison. Both the latter components also contribute to energy intake without providing commensurate amounts of essential nutrients.

These principles involved in choosing a healthy diet in an affluent country are well known, and not difficult to apply. However, at least two categories of people need more help than is offered by these general principles. In one category are children entering primary school at age five years who are already overweight for their height. It is a mistake to try to get young children to lose weight, since weight loss is always associated with a slowing of the normal increase in height, but it is also a mistake to ignore the situation in the hope that the child will grow out of it. An average child aged five years is approximately 1.1 m tall and weights 18 kg, and by 12 years is 1.5 m tall and weights 40 kg. A child who is 4 kg overweight at five years is probably on the 90th centile of weight for height, and is very likely to become an obese teenager. However, if this child can gain height normally over the next seven years, and gain only 18 kg in weight instead of the average 22 kg, the result should be a child who enters the teen years at a normal weight for height. To achieve this control of weight gain in overweight children entering primary school will require the intelligent co-operation of parents, teachers, school nurses and caterers, and the children themselves. However, I believe that the benefits to the child would be very great, so it is worthwhile to try to obtain this co-operation.

The other category of people who need special help are adults who are already overweight. There are many commercial slimming clubs which vie for trade, some of which make unduly optimistic claims for the rate of weight loss which can be achieved on their regimen. When customers fail to achieve the advertised results, they assume that they must have a particularly refractory metabolism and are liable to be duped by charlatans advertising magic cures which are incompatible with the well-tested laws of thermodynamics. Traditionally, obesity has not been a prime target for health educators in the UK, so there is no authoritative advice available to counteract the unscientific nonsense. I believe obesity should be given the importance it deserves as a public health problem.[30]

This brief review has concentrated on the diseases which relate to the diet in affluent countries. Some would argue that eating disorders such as anorexia nervosa and the less easily recognized syndrome of bulimia nervosa also fall under the heading of diseases of diet in affluent countries, but these are primarily disorders of perception of body image. People who suffer from anorexia say that they started on a regimen of self-starvation because they were only trying to rescue themselves from the dangers of obesity, but when it is possible to check the weight status of the patient before the onset of anorexia it is rarely above the normal range. The syndromes of anorexia and bulimia nervosa serve to remind us that we should be discriminating about advice on weight control. The message is not that everyone should lose weight, but that everyone needs to be vigilant about avoiding excessive weight gain; it is an important difference.

Summary

The well-intentioned efforts of food technologists have brought to the populations of affluent countries a food supply which is far safer, more abundant and varied than that obtainable by the average person in poorer countries. Although this situation brings many benefits, it also brings problems, most of which relate to the difficulty in regulating energy intake when the food offered is palatable, varied and novel. The sophistication of the food consumers must match that of the food providers, since physiological regulation is inadequate for the task.

Maintenance of a desirable body weight, and an adequate intake of fresh fruit, vegetables and dietary fibre, is perfectly possible in an affluent country, but it requires conscious effort. If food intake is guided by our untutored instincts, we are likely to get too fat and to choose a diet which tends to accelerate the rate of aging of our tissues, thereby rendering ourselves more liable to the diseases which characterize the populations of affluent countries.

NOTES

1 Secretary of State for Health (1991) *The Health of the Nation*, London, HMSO.
2 Waterlow, J. C. (1989) 'Diet in the classical period of Greece and Rome', *European Journal of Clinical Nutrition* 43 (Supplement 2), 3–12.
3 Davidson, S., Passmore, R. and Brock, J. F. (1973) *Human Nutrition and Dietetics*, 5th edn, Edinburgh, Churchill Livingstone, p. 246.
4 Lane-Petter, W. (1970) 'Do laboratory animals like eating?', *Proceeding of the Nutrition Society* 29, 335–8.
5 Booth, D. A., Lee, M. and McAleavey, C. (1976) 'Acquired sensory control of satiation in man', *British Journal of Psychology* 67, 137–47.
6 Rolls, B. J., Van Duijvenvoorde, P. M. and Rolls, E. T. (1984) 'Pleasantness changes and food intake in a varied four-course meal', *Appetite* 5, 337–48.
7 Boswell, J. (1782) 'The applause of the Jury 1781–1785', in I. R. Lustig and F. A. Pottle (eds) (1982) *The Private Papers of James Boswell*, London, Heinemann.

8 Behnke, A. R., Feen, B. G. and Welham, W. C. (1942) 'The specific gravity of healthy men: body weight and volume as an index of obesity', *Journal of the American Medical Association* 118, 495–8.
9 Johnson, M. L., Burke, B. S. and Meyer, J. (1956) 'The relative importance of inactivity and overeating in the energy balance of obese high school girls', *American Journal of Clinical Nutrition* 4, 37–44.
10 Keys, A., Menotti, A., Aravanis, C., Blackburn, H., Djordevic, B. S., Buzina, R., Dontas, A. S., Fidanza, F., Karvonen, M. J., Kimura, N., Mohacek, I., Nedeljkovic, S., Puddu, V., Punsar, S., Taylor, H. L., Conti, S., Kromhout, D. and Toshima, H. (1984) 'The seven countries study: 2289 deaths in 15 years', *Preventive Medicine* 13, 141–54.
11 Garrow, J. S. and Webster, J. (1985) 'Quetelet's index (W/H^2) as a measure of fatness', *International Journal of Obesity* 9, 147–53.
12 Garrow, J. S. (1988) *Obesity and Related Diseases*, London, Churchill Livingstone.
13 Folsom, A. R., Burke, G. L., Byers, C. L., Hutchinson, R. G., Heiss, G., Flack, J. M., Jacobs, D. R. and Cann, B. (1991) 'Implications of obesity for cardiovascular disease in blacks: the CARDIA and ARIC studies', *American Journal of Clinical Nutrition* 53, 1604S–11S.
14 Hubert, H. B. (1984) 'The nature of the relationship between obesity and cardiovascular disease', *International Journal of Cardiology* 6, 268–74.
15 Jeanrenaud, B. (1991) 'Neuroendocrinology and evolutionary aspects of experimental obesity', in Y. Oomura, S. Tarui, S. Inoue and T. Shimazu (eds) *Progress in Obesity Research 1990*, London, John Libbey, pp. 409–21.
16 Sims, E. A. H., Danforth, E. Jr, Horton, E. S., Bray, G. A., Glennon, J. A. and Salans, L. B. (1973) 'Endocrine and metabolic effects of experimental obesity in man', *Recent Progress in Hormone Research* 29, 457–9.
17 Shaper, A. G. (1988) *Coronary Heart Disease, Risks and Reasons*, London, Current Medical Literature.
18 Modan, M., Halkin, H., Almog, S., Lusky, A., Eshkol, A., Shefi, M., Shitrit, A. and Fuchs, Z. (1985) 'Hyperinsulinaemia: a link between hypertension, obesity and glucose intolerance', *Journal of Clinical Investigation* 75, 809–17.
19 Førde, O. H., Thelle, D. S., Arnesen, E. and Mjos, O. D. (1986) 'Distribution of high density lipoprotein cholesterol according to relative body weight, cigarette smoking and leisure time physical activity', *Acta Medica Scandinavica* 219, 167–71.
20 Garfinkel, L. (1985) 'Overweight and cancer', *Annals of Internal Medicine* 103, 1034–6.
21 Reuben, A., Maton, P. N., Murphy, G. M. and Dowling, R. H. (1985) 'Bile lipid secretion in obese and non-obese individuals with and without gallstones', *Clinical Science* 69, 71–9.
22 Nomura, F., Ohnishi, K., Satomura, Y., Ohtsuki, T., Fukungaga, K., Honda, M., Ema, M., Tohyama, T., Sugita, S., Saito, M., Iida, S. and Okuda, K. (1986) 'Liver function in moderate obesity – study in 534 moderately obese subjects among 4613 male company employees', *International Journal of Obesity* 10, 349–54.
23 Rissanen, A., Heliovaara, M., Knekt, P., Reunanen, A., Aromaa, A. and Maatela, J. (1990) 'Risk of disability and mortality due to overweight in a Finnish population', *British Medical Journal* 301, 835–6.

24 Elkeles, R. S. (1991) 'Lipids in non-insulin dependent diabetes: a case for treatment?', *Proceedings of the Royal Society of Medicine* 84, 393–4.

25 Borkan, G. A., Sparrow, D., Wisniewski, C. and Vokonas, P. S. (1986) 'Body weight and coronary heart disease risk: patterns of risk factor change associated with long-term weight change', *American Journal of Epidemiology* 124, 410–19.

26 Hubert, H. B. (1986) 'The importance of obesity in the development of coronary risk factors and disease: the epidemiological evidence', *Annual Reviews of Public Health* 7, 493–502.

27 MacMahon, S. M., Macdonald, G. J., Bernstein, L., Andrews, G. and Blacket, R. B. (1985) 'A randomised controlled trial of weight reduction and metoprolol in the treatment of hypertension in young overweight patients', *Clinical and Experimental Pharmacology and Physiology* 12, 267–71.

28 Rosenbaum, S., Skinner, R. K., Knight, I. B. and Garrow, J. S. (1985) 'A survey of heights and weights of adults in Great Britain', *Annals of Human Biology* 12, 115–27.

29 Gregory, J., Foster, K., Tyler, H. and Wiseman, M. (1990) *The Dietary and Nutritional Survey of British Adults*, London, HMSO.

30 Garrow, J. S. (1991) 'Importance of obesity', *British Medical Journal* 303, 704–6.

5

Not Enough Food: Malnutrition and Famine

Philip Payne

The main emphasis of this chapter will be to give an account of the current state of understanding of the biology of food deprivation and to show how a lack of adequate nutrition acts in combination with other aspects of a poor environment, in particular with infectious diseases, to produce a range of different kinds of health problems. However, all scientists like to think that their contributions to understanding how the world works will have an immediate impact on human welfare. An underlying theme, therefore, will be about the way nutritional science has been applied to defining the nature and extent of health and social problems during the twentieth century and how, from time to time, new understanding has led to the need for reappraisal of the nature and extent of those problems.

Anyone attempting that kind of analysis faces a perilous voyage. The problem is that, unlike many other diseases, malnutrition comes not only in a variety of forms, but with a whole range of intensities and outcomes. Quantifying malnutrition, however, requires us to use some clearly defined criteria to identify who is malnourished and for what reason, and to estimate how many are affected.

It seems evident that this is essential not only for choosing policies or relevant interventions, but also for raising social awareness and mobilizing political support for change. However, there are quite sharp divisions amongst academics and the members of the various professional groups involved about the correct tactical and conceptual approaches. At the risk of some oversimplification, these differences of viewpoint can be described as a polarization of positions between those who wish always to err on the side of including as many as possible in the category of malnourished – the malnutrition 'maximalists' – and the malnutrition 'minimalists', whose main concern is with accurately identifying those people who are certainly, rather than possibly, suffering from the effects of a poor diet.

If we adopt broader, more inclusive criteria, we are likely to end up with much larger numbers who may be affected in some way and to some degree by food deprivation, but with less precision about the nature of their circumstances or the causes. If, on the other hand, our criteria for identifying the malnourished are stringent and highly specific, we may end up with a comparatively small number, but a correspondingly sharper focus on the social and environmental context within which malnutrition occurs.

Both approaches have their advocates, not only amongst nutritionists, but also amongst economists and social scientists, many of whom have come to believe, in my view somewhat mistakenly, that nutritional science can provide not only more precise, but also more objective criteria for identifying the poor than can the techniques of their own disciplines.

The minimalists on the whole seek to avoid exaggeration of the extent of the problems and are concerned to secure political support for the improvement of those who are worst off. In terms of action, they are often inclined towards gradual implementation and extension of targeted interventions, or with improving the efficiency of existing programmes. The maximalists, on the other hand, want to generate the greatest possible level of moral outrage, followed by the widest possible inclusion of beneficiaries of any remedial action. To that end, the scientific definition of malnutrition must be such as to capture the widest possible degree of social consensus on the need for change.

Both approaches deserve respect, but also hold dangers, not least of which is the risk of becoming engaged in bitter controversy! The maximalists accuse the minimalists of 'talking down' the problems of food deprivation. The minimalists accuse the maximalists of being more concerned with arousing popular support than with efficiency and consistency of implementation.

My own position tends towards the minimalist side, perhaps more from scientific caution than for any other reason: over the years, so many 'discoveries' have been followed by recantations, and so many expensive trials of nutrition programmes have turned out in the end to have had little or no effect. I believe it is premature for nutritionists to claim an understanding of more than a small fraction of the range of conditions of poor health which might have dietary causes.

Counting the Numbers of the Malnourished

Perhaps the first and, in the UK, the best-known person to use nutritional standards to support a minimalist assessment of the extent of poverty, was Benjamin Seebohm Rowntree, in his study of poverty in the city of York, published in 1901.[1] Rowntree was well aware of the danger of having his work dismissed by the political establishment of the time as lacking objectivity. Accordingly, he drew a precise distinction between primary and secondary poverty. Primary poverty was the poverty of those families whose incomes were insufficient to provide the bare necessities of physical efficiency, no matter how wisely and carefully their incomes were spent. Secondary poverty, on the other hand, characterized those families whose state of physical health was also poor, despite their having incomes above the threshold of primary poverty. Rowntree described the condition of life of people living at the threshold of survival in the following terms:

> A family living on the scale allowed for in this estimate must never spend a penny on rail fare or omnibus. They must never go into the country unless they walk. They must never purchase a halfpenny newspaper or spend a penny to buy a ticket for a popular concert. They must write no letters to absent children, for they cannot afford to pay the postage. They must never contribute anything to their church or chapel, or give any help to a neighbour which costs them money.
>
> They cannot save, nor can they join a sick club or Trade Union, because they cannot pay the necessary subscriptions. The children must have no pocket money for dolls, marbles or sweets. The father must smoke no tobacco and drink no beer. The mother must buy no pretty clothes for herself, or for her children, the character of the family wardrobe as for the family diet being governed by the regulation, 'Nothing must be bought but that which is absolutely necessary for the maintenance of physical health and what must be bought must be of the plainest description'. Should a child fall ill it must be attended by the parish doctor: should it die it must be buried by the parish. Finally, the wage earner must never be absent from his work for a single day.

Adding, 'that if any of these conditions are broken, the extra expenditure is met, and can only be met, by limiting the diet; or in other words by sacrificing *physical efficiency*'. He went on to establish the composition and cost of a weekly shopping basket of food, sufficient to meet what were at that time considered to be minimally adequate nutritional criteria. On this basis, he reported that some 10 per cent of families were living below that threshold, in a state of primary poverty. His estimates of the cost revealed that if physical efficiency were not to be sacrificed, these families had no alternative but to spend a proportion of their income on food similar to the 80 per cent expended by the poorest families in the Third World today.

Rowntree's fear of being accused of vague emotional sympathy for those whose poverty was due to their own weakness of character, was well founded in the general attitudes of the day: a *Times* leader referred to his description of primary poverty as 'fairly comfortable'!

At the time, Rowntree's work contributed greatly to a better understanding of poverty: especially that many of the poor were so totally constrained by their limited incomes that they were in no position to improve their own condition by wiser budgeting. Sadly, as seems to have happened often in the past, Rowntree's threshold of survival was reinterpreted as a standard of adequacy by the British Medical Association (BMA) committee

Table 5.1 Percentage of global population estimated to be living on inadequate dietary energy intakes

Year of estimate	*Percent of population hungry*	*Source of estimate*
1963	10–15	FAO
1965	55	WB
1970	19	FAO
1970	40	WB
1973	25	FAO
1980	15	FAO
1980	34	WB

of 1934, which had been asked to assist the government to establish a scientific basis for the level of unemployment relief. The chairman of the scientific committee, Sir John Boyd Orr, later became the first Director General of the Food and Agriculture Organization (FAO). It was his statement in the early 1950s, that two-thirds of the population of the developing world were doomed to a life of hunger and want, that became the first of many 'maximalist' analyses of the global food and nutrition situation.

This kind of assessment has been repeated several times during the past 40 years, not only by the FAO,[2–5] but also by the World Bank (WB),[6,7] in both cases using much the same sources of statistics, but with different and, over time, increasingly elaborate technical and mathematical methods.

In addition to the implications of these numbers for health and survival, continued widespread hunger has been suggested as an explanation for the slow rate of economic and social development of some of the poorer Third World countries.

I believe that this essentially Malthusian hypothesis, that hunger is the single direct cause not only of most human illness, but also of people's apparent inability to overcome their own poverty, is probably not correct, or at least, that it is not the most useful way of understanding the problems of the developing world. Before giving reasons in support of this, I want to anticipate any accusation that in doing so, I am in some way discounting the importance of taking action to alleviate hunger and food deprivation where these are known to exist.

The existence of hunger is manifest to anyone who attends to the news media. However, it is the persistence of any amount of avoidable suffering which is morally objectionable. A global rate of malnutrition of 30 per cent of the population would certainly pose massive resource problems, but 3 per cent would, in terms of human values, be just as unacceptable. In addition to this, it will become clear later that, far from 'talking down' the needs of the poor of the Third World for a fairer share of the benefits of economic development, I shall be suggesting that a genuine effort to accelerate the rate of improvement of nutrition-related health will require a much more fundamental redistribution, not only of physical resources, but also of people's entitlement and access to them, than would be involved solely in improving the distribution of food.

There are three kinds of reason for rejecting the 'hungry world' hypothesis. The first two are methodological. The food standards against which consumption levels have been compared were originally intended to represent the average needs of healthy populations – they were indeed based on the observed intakes of such groups. It is hardly surprising to find that up to 50 per cent of any population will be found to be eating less than such an average – a flippant dismissal perhaps, but one with more than a grain of truth. Secondly, the data on consumption – at least, the only data currently available – are aggregated to the level of whole countries and are derived from records of annual production, together with imports and exports of food. For technical reasons, these tend to be biased on the low side, particularly in the poorer countries, which have the worst statistical services.

Perhaps the most telling arguments come from the improved understanding that has been gained over the past decade or so about food requirements, in particular about the capacity of humans to adapt to different levels of consumption, the significance of different body sizes and the importance of infectious disease as a contributory cause of malnutrition.

The Alien Ecologist's View

There is something of an inherent paradox in the 'hungry world' hypothesis. Imagine for a moment the response of a visitor from a different world – perhaps an ecologist – asked to comment on the biological success of the human species. The alien would be likely to say that, in comparison with other species of comparable body size, humans seem to have achieved a greater total biomass (i.e. the sum of the body weights of all individuals now alive). Moreover, in recent times, this has been combined not only with a rapid rate of increase of numbers, but also with a continually rising proportion of all individuals born, who survive to contribute to future generations. It would go on to say that this simply could not be the case if a substantial proportion of the human population were constantly experiencing the detrimental effects of hunger and famine. Either the data which seem to show this must be wrong, or the word 'hunger' has not been defined in biological terms. It might, however, go on to add a cautionary

Table 5.2 A classification of nutritional states

	Stress		
	Malnutrition	*Undernutrition*	*Infections*
	Deficiencies of:	Low intake of food energy	Virus
	Iodine		Bacterium
	Iron		
Strain	Vitamin A		Plasmodium
	Vitamin C		
	.		
	.		
	Protein ?		Microfilarium
	.		
	~ 42 kinds		etc.
Functional Capacity	Adaptation/ Reduction	Adaptation/ Reduction	Reduced
		Weight loss	Weight loss
Body size		Height growth reduced	Height growth reduced
Survival	Reduced	Reduced/Increased	Reduced

rider, that because global population has not so far been constrained by any Malthusian 'positive check', it is not a sufficient reason for assuming that it will never happen.

The Biology of Hunger

Let us first consider a very simple classification of the different types of malnutrition. The columns of table 5.2 describe a number of 'stresses' that can occur in individuals as a result of dietary insufficiencies of different kinds or of the indirect nutritional effects of infectious diseases. The rows describe the different types of 'strains', which are the responses made by the body in countering those stresses. This idea of various states of nutrition (i.e. strains) as graded responses to different types and magnitudes of environmental stresses has been used in order to counteract the common tendency to think of malnutrition as analogous to the distinct states of 'illness', as opposed to 'health', which result for example from either having or not having a virus infection.

The word 'stress', in common usage, generally connotes something unpleasant (it is in fact a contracted form of 'distress'): at best to be avoided, at worst a threat to life or happiness. To an engineer or biologist, however, the word simply describes the forces or interactions between systems and their external environments. An animal, a piece of machinery, a colony of birds or a building are all constantly exposed to the stresses of various external forces applied to them, whether mechanical or otherwise. Thus, a building is stressed by the weight of its contents, or by the pressure of wind, or by the shock wave of an earthquake.

Other kinds of words are needed to describe how systems adjust to applied stresses. Beams bend, whole buildings tilt, animals hibernate, colonies migrate. The engineer uses these responses to quantify the 'strain' in a system and will characterize the way a structure handles different levels of stress in terms of stress–strain relationships. It is the nature and magnitude of these various adjustments or strains, the symptoms of which, taken together, constitute the overall reaction to stress (in a plant or animal) which, together with knowledge about the side-effects and sequelae of the component adjustments, finally determine whether we assess the outcome as good or bad.

Kinds of Nutritional Stress

An important distinction is to be made between undernutrition and malnutrition. The stress of undernutrition is simply that of starvation: having insufficient energy in the diet to meet the requirements of the body for maintaining its physical and chemical functions and to supply the energy needed for movement, doing physical work and, in young individuals, for growing. Malnutrition, strictly speaking, is the result of eating the wrong kinds of foods, that is, an unbalanced mixture of the chemical constituents of food, resulting in relative deficiencies or surpluses of some of these. It is obvious that either of these types of stress can be of variable intensity and duration.

Table 5.2 shows a third form of stress, that which is influenced by an additional cause, infectious disease. Diet and disease interact in such a complex and mutually reinforcing way that it is frequently difficult – often impossible – to distinguish either one as the primary cause of stress. An infection can result in loss of appetite and hence initiate undernutrition; it can also result in the depletion of body stores of specific nutrients and hence malnutrition. Dietary deficiencies, on the other hand, can reduce the effectiveness of response of the body's immune system, making infection more likely and increasing its severity. In these ways, either diet or disease can act as initial causes of stress and both can interact in a mutually reinforcing way. Since poverty generally results in people having frequently to cope with coinciding food and disease problems, it is impossible to overemphasize the importance of this interaction for any attempt to comprehend the nature and magnitude of the impact of global hunger.

Malnutrition

Table 5.2 suggests that there are 42 different kinds of malnutrition. However, as admirers of Douglas Adams might suspect, that number was chosen simply to suggest that there are a large number, at least 40 or so distinct chemical elements, types of molecules and groups of compounds, all of which must be present in the diets of humans in order to avoid some loss of functional capacity. Out of this large number of possible causes of deficiency disease, four have been recognized for a very long time: iodine, iron and vitamins C and A. Indeed, the dire results of vitamin C deficiency (scurvy) have been known for centuries. In 1753, the Scottish physician, James Lind, published his *Treatise on the Scurvy*. This showed that a disease which was frequently fatal for sailors on long voyages could be prevented simply by a daily ration of vegetables or lemon juice. The prescription was so effective that, whereas Anson in 1740 had failed to circumnavigate the globe largely because half his crew had died of scurvy, Cook succeeded in 1774 without the loss of a single man from the disease.

Despite this very practical success, Lind's theory about how it worked was not popular. He believed that scurvy was caused by the absence of something in the diet – an idea that seems perfectly reasonable today. Contemporary medical scientists, however, found it totally unacceptable. They 'knew' that diseases were caused by the presence of something bad – a poison, a miasma (or later on a bacterium). Lind, who tried without success to produce scurvy by deliberate experiment in groups of volunteers, finally lost faith in his own idea and died disillusioned. Had he been alive today, Lind might have been cheered by the news that the 'missing' molecule has been identified, but depressed again to learn that, despite that knowledge and understanding, people are still dying of scurvy, for example Somalian refugees confined in camps in Ethiopia, nominally under the protection of the United Nations (UN).

The other three, iron, iodine and vitamin A, are now sometimes referred to collectively as the 'supernutrients', and the effects of lack of them as 'hidden hunger', on the grounds that the people who suffer are unaware of the cause. Symptoms of deficiency are certainly very common in many of the poorer developing countries. Table 5.3 shows some recent estimates

Table 5.3 Numbers of people 'at risk' and with definite symptoms of malnutrition

	Iodine		*Vitamin A*		*Iron*
Region	*Present*	*At risk*	*Present*	*At risk*	*At risk*
Africa	39	150	1.3	18	206
Americas	30	55	0.1	2	94
S. E. Asia	100	280	10.0	138	616
Europe	26	105	1.0	13	176
W. Pacific	30	405	1.4	19	1058
Total	225	995	13.8	190	2150

published by the World Health Organization.[8] In this table, an important distinction is made between those people in whom definite symptoms of deficiency are present, and those who are considered to be at risk, because although not visibly suffering, their circumstances of life are similar to those who are.

The UN and some other, but not all, relief agencies, advise the governments of countries in these regions to take a short cut to better health by using technical means – tablets, injections, fortification of salt, etc. – to treat the symptoms and continue to distribute these nutrients for as long as may be necessary, in order to prevent recurrence.

Others argue that, although these substances themselves are cheap, the same cannot be said of the resources needed for the transport, distribution management and supervision of such mass interventions. These 'human resources' are very scarce in poor countries. Indeed, their scarcity is as much a part of the poverty of a nation as is a lack of money. Programmes for distributing micronutrients may therefore be mounted at the expense of other things, some of which might contribute as much or more to social or economic improvement in the longer term, thereby rendering such continuous treatment unnecessary. Whether preventing 'hidden hunger' turns out to be any easier than preventing the more conventional kind remains to be seen.

Undernutrition

This kind of stress, namely, insufficient food energy content to match the amount expended, probably comes closest to what people have in mind

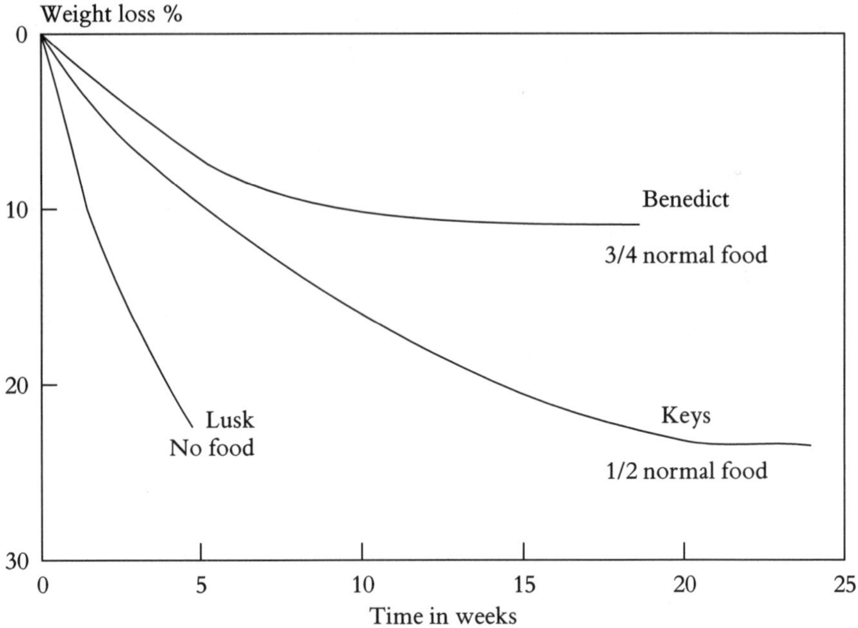

Figure 5.1 Body weight loss during fasting.

when they talk about world hunger. However, the word hunger has no scientific definition and there are no agreed methods for measuring it. Moreover, according to circumstance, it has more than one common implication: for some people, at some times, a signal of desperation; for others, an expression of keen healthy appetite. Compare, for example, the likely implications of a complaint of 'hunger' by a child in an Ethiopian peasant family with those of a similar plea made to almost any Western parent!

Less problematic is starvation, the meaning of which is sustained undernutrition: a continuing deficit of energy intake below energy expenditure. Because the first law of thermodynamics operates for people as well as for machines, this must mean a continuous loss of body weight, ultimately leading to death. Figure 5.1 shows the results of three undernutrition experiments carried out on human volunteers at various times during the past century.

The curves are of the percentage of body weight lost and the names beside each are those of the experimenters, not the subjects, who were all young male college students. Lusk[9] studied total starvation, giving his subjects only water, terminating the trials when it was considered too dangerous to continue. This was generally close to the biblical estimate of 40 days and 40 nights. Keys[10] and Benedict[11] started by measuring how much food energy their subjects normally ate and then gave them either 1/2 or 3/4 of that amount. In both these experiments, the subjects lost weight until the point at which their bodies only needed that amount of energy they were being given in order to maintain themselves, at which point they were, technically, no longer starving. Keys' subjects were allowed to reduce their level of physical activity and finally moved about very little. Benedict's were encouraged to maintain their normal pattern of work and leisure. Neither Lusk's nor Keys' subjects had any sensation of hunger after the first two days of the experiment, that is, whatever that sensation means, it is a relatively short-term experience.

The point of this description is to illustrate that undernutrition due to food being given at a reduced but fixed level must be understood as having two phases. During the first, energy intake is less than energy expenditure and the first law of thermodynamics dictates that either body weight and/or physical activity must decline until the second phase when, because of the counteracting strain (reduced body weight), the balance between the two is again restored; in other words, we must distinguish the process of undernutrition from the condition of having been undernourished. This seemingly fine distinction becomes very important when it is realized that the ways in which people have tried to estimate the extent of hunger have all depended on calculations of the numbers for whom food energy available is apparently less than the energy they require (i.e. their estimated energy expenditure). Hence, if the numbers in table 5.1, for example, were to be taken at face value, they would need to be thought of as the percentage of the world population which is currently experiencing the process of undernutrition or starvation, that is, people who are continuously either losing weight, or progressively becoming less physically active, or both. In addition, the numbers must exclude those people who have already lost weight and/or had to reduce their physical activity to the point where intake balances expenditure, that is, those who have already been through the process of starvation. As our imaginary alien visitor pointed out, all of which would have to be happening along with rates of population growth which, in the poorest countries, typically cause a doubling of numbers every 20 years.

In addition to the evidence of high fertility rates, it seems likely that in populations in which between 20 and 50 per cent of people were in the process of undernutrition, mortality rates would be high and rising over time. Tables 5.4 and 5.5 show that the reverse is the case. The world average crude mortality rate (i.e. deaths at all ages and for both sexes) now stands at 9 for every 1000 persons per year, corresponding to a life expectancy at birth of 65 years. We need to remember, of course, that some age groups are more vulnerable than others to the effects of all three kinds of

Table 5.4 Crude death rates by region and decline over 23 years

Region	*Deaths per 1000 in 1965*	*Deaths per 1000 in 1988*	*Rate of decrease (% per year)*	*Population (millions)*
World	14	9	1.6	5210
Sub-Saharan Africa	23	15	1.5	480
East Asia	11	7	1.6	1520
South Asia	20	11	2.0	1130
S. America & Caribbean	12	7	1.8	420
Mid-income Countries	15	10	1.4	4052
Severely Indebted	12	8	1.4	554
High-income Countries	10	9	0.4	830

Table 5.5 Infant mortality by region and decline over 23 years

Region	*Deaths per 1000 under 1yr in 1965*	*Deaths per 1000 under 1yr in 1988*	*Rate of decrease (% per year)*	*Population (millions)*
World	92	54	1.8	5210
Sub-Saharan Africa	157	107	1.4	480
East Asia	95	35	2.7	1520
South Asia	147	95	1.5	1130
S. America & Caribbean	94	50	2.0	420
Mid-income Countries	117	65	1.9	4052
Severely Indebted	93	51	1.9	554
High-income Countries	25	9	2.8	830

nutrition-related stress, but even amongst the youngest age groups average death rates are falling, as table 5.5 shows.

It seems likely that much of the remaining differences in average life expectancy between regions is due to these much larger differences in mortality in early life. In fact, table 5.4 shows that in the high-income countries, the rate of increase of average life expectancy is beginning to fall, reflecting approach to the biological maximum. This is particularly marked in the case of populations such as that of Japan, which now has a mean life expectancy at birth of 78 years, possibly close to the maximum achievable, short of the use of genetic engineering to manipulate the process of senescence.

Undernutrition, Body Size and Adaptation

It must be clear by now that, whatever the real significance of the numbers in table 5.1, they cannot be a measure of the extent of active starvation. However, we noted in passing that, in any case, they probably by definition exclude individuals who have survived and adjusted to that process by becoming smaller or less active. It would be very reasonable to describe such people as undernourished. The question is how could we identify them? Certainly, we cannot do it by measuring their energy intakes, since we should simply find that, whilst low, they were sufficient to match their expenditures. The problem is that two other kinds of people will also be found to have lower than average food intakes. First, there will be those who are smaller than average size for other reasons: because of their genes, because they have recently been ill, or because they have never made up for interruptions of growth when they were young children (permanent growth stunting is a common feature of the first one or two years of life in impoverished populations, as will be discussed later). Second, there will be individuals with low expenditures of energy on work because of un- or underemployment.

One of the ideas which has generated most passionate dispute between the 'maximalist' and 'minimalist' schools of thought is the proposition that poor people might in some way be said to be able to adapt to an inadequate diet by becoming smaller or by working less. Faced with that proposition, social and public health scientists have generally been unwilling to use the word 'adaptation' on the grounds that it seems to imply some kind of success (even if only in a biological sense). 'We', they say, should not be willing to describe a human condition as successful when it is, in fact, the outcome of a process which 'succeeds' through the 'barest survival' of individuals. Notwithstanding that reluctance, however, in the ensuing discussion I shall use the word adaptation in its evolutionary sense. That is to say, in relation to responses to nutritional stress likely to have contributed in the past to 'fitness', in the sense of increased or maintained probability, given the stress of survival through the period, of producing and supporting viable offspring. Adaptations are normally to a new maintainable steady state (until senescence); conservative of functions under threat; and sometimes, but not necessarily, reversible. Of course, there will be limits to the extent to which a person can adapt through reducing either body weight or energy expenditure. Looking back to figure 5.1, somewhere in between the levels of food restriction chosen by Benedict and by Keys there is a point on the weight-loss scale below which functional capacity is compromised through loss of muscle mass, damage to other tissues, loss of capacity to combat the effects of infections or other insults. The problem, which is so far unresolved, is how to identify that point.

What we shall undoubtedly find, as in most adaptive changes which have been established through the process of natural selection, will be that there is a set of advantages contributing to fitness in some circumstances, together with a set of counteracting disadvantages.

It is the net balance or trade-off between the advantages and disadvantages of, for example, becoming smaller which decides the success or failure of that strategy of adaptation. However, this will always apply to a particular context. If we conclude that the extent of hunger is to be measured by the numbers of people who suffer harm of some kind because their capacity to adapt has been exceeded, this is likely always to need an examination of particular circumstances rather than the application of some global criteria for acceptable minimum values of height or weight. For the moment, the best that can be done is to describe some of the good and the bad consequences to people of having to become smaller in response to nutritional stress.

Perhaps the most obvious advantage is that food needs are less. This is most striking if we look at the saving of energy over time. The first part of table 5.6 shows the body weight from six months of age up to adulthood of an average European girl. The lower part of the table shows that of a girl typical of many rural Asian populations. A comparison of the weights shows them diverging some time between six months and one year. In each case, below the values for weight are those for the three components of daily energy requirements: (1) maintenance (the energy cost of just staying alive, with no energy used for physical activity or growth); (2) growth (the energy needed to synthesize and store new tissue); and (3) activity (the energy cost of moving the body and other objects around). The table shows the daily energy requirement of each girl, which is the sum of these three components. The next row of values is for the total energy needed, added up for all the days the two girls have lived up to the particular ages at the top of each column. The two rows at the bottom of the table show the amounts of energy 'saved' as a result of the smaller size of the Asian as compared with the European girl at each particular age.

The daily savings are simply the differences between the daily rates. While the children are very young, these are relatively small amounts; at one year, the difference is 80 Kcal a day. Not much of an immediate saving to the individual, even less to her whole family which, taken together, is likely to have a daily requirement of between 8 and 10 thousand Kcal. However, as the last row in the table shows, the cumulative differences, that is, the daily savings added up over the 25 years, are very substantial; by the time she reaches adulthood, the Asian has used more than 4 million Kcals less energy than the European, which is sufficient to feed another younger sister up to the age of ten.

So, if being small can have its advantages, what about the penalties? To answer that question, we first need to consider in more detail how the adjustment in size takes place, in particular during the process of growth.

Table 5.6 Saving of energy resulting from reduced growth rate

	Body size and energy needs			
Age (years)	0.5	1	10	25
European girl				
Weight (kg)	7.2	9.5	35.2	57
Calories per day	660	990	1910	2220
Lifetime total	94 900	245 500	5166 600	16 472 000
Asian girl				
Weight (kg)	7.2	9	22.5	43
Calories per day	660	910	1310	1742
Lifetime total	94 900	238 200	4036 000	12 390 000
Energy saving				
Calories per day	0	80	600	478
Lifetime	0	7300	1130 600	4082 000

Source: Gray, A. (ed.) (1993) *World Health and Disease*, Milton Keynes, Open University Press.

Nutrition, Infection and Growth

If there is one commonly held idea about nutritionists, it is that they are people who are skilled in assessing the 'nutritional status' of a child simply by weighing it and measuring its height or arm circumference. It will come as a shock to many people to learn that there is a rapidly growing consensus that the more or less indiscriminate connection of smallness with the notion of malnutrition has been, in the words of at least one highly respected expert, 'an unfortunate accident of history'.[12] One of the starting points for this revolution in thinking was an attempt in the early 1980s to make a rigorous evaluation of child feeding programmes. Briefly, the verdict was that when these were directed at children between the ages of weaning up to six years, they had had almost no effect on growth, or at any rate very much less than would have been expected.

Growth is known to be adversely affected by the third kind of food-related stress shown in table 5.2, that is, that created by the interaction between under- or malnutrition and infectious diseases. This can be particularly severe during the later stages of intra-uterine life, together with the first few years or so after birth. Up to about the age of two years, when in pre-industrial societies weaning is complete, there is, however, also a capacity to 'catch up' on any lost growth, provided the stress is reversed and provided there is sufficient food and parental care to support faster growth and larger size. However, as the end of this critical period is approached, the ability to fully recover is reduced. The result is that, if a child suffers repeated episodes of stress through and beyond the second year of life, it will end up with an accumulated shortfall in both height and weight which is permanent. Not only that, the deficit is 'carried over' into the next phase of life in the form of a modified set of 'instructions' for the mechanisms by which the body achieves its final adult size. These altered instructions, even in the absence of further stress, result in an adult shorter in height (and correspondingly lower in weight) than he or she would have been without the stresses during infancy. It has been found that, although this process of growth 'stunting' can be reduced by improving the health environment of mothers and infants, relatively little can be done to reverse any growth deficits remaining at a later stage, which explains why food distribution programmes targeted at children older than two years have so little effect on growth.

The curve of growth in height shown in figure 5.2 illustrates this process in a diagrammatic way. A girl whose length as a baby follows the average of the normal range (the smooth curve labelled 50th centile) suffers a series of setbacks to growth and manages to catch up again at first, but after the age of two years further illness causes growth to fall away towards the lower end of the normal range (the dotted curve labelled 3rd centile), and the girl finally becomes an adult whose height growth finishes at the lower end of the normal range.

Infectious diseases of early childhood, such as diarrhoeal or respiratory tract infections, not only affect growth directly through the toxins they produce in the body, but also act indirectly through reduced appetite. If growth is severely affected, from whatever cause, there may also be damage to the immune systems which defend the child from infections, increasing the likelihood of further severe illness. Thus, whatever the nature of the initiating event, disease or inadequate food, the outcome is likely to be the same: a self-reinforcing sequence of growth checks, with any remaining deficit in height after about two years being followed by a lifelong pattern of smallness.

This description of the process of becoming small as one which has its major impact in very early life, but which then leads on to a more or less irreversible state of relative smallness in later life, has several important implications for our general inquiry into the nature and extent of hunger. First, it means that we should be very cautious about using measurements

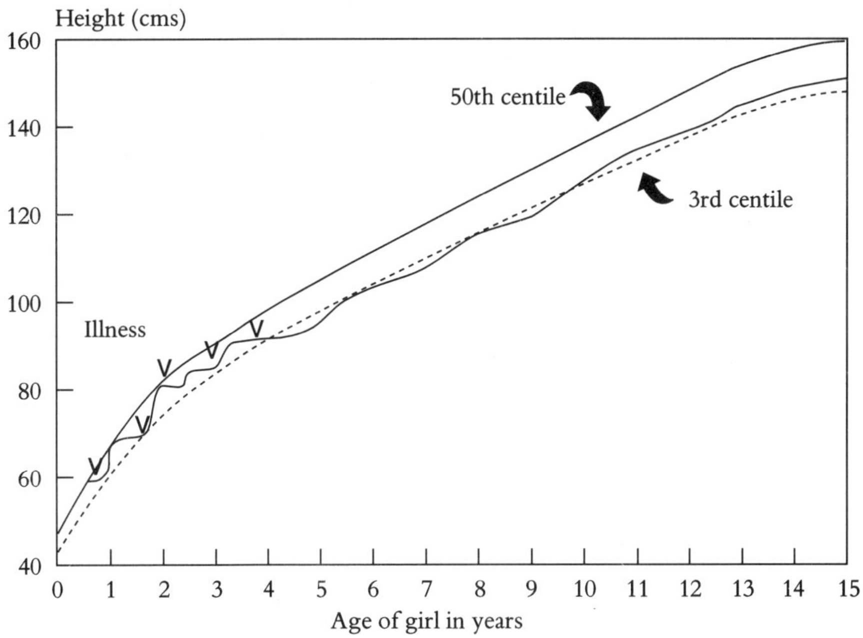

Figure 5.2 Effect of early illness on height growth. (*Source*: Gray, A., 1993, ed., *World Health and Disease*, Milton Keynes, Open University Press.)

of the current body sizes of adult populations as a means of assessing current levels of nutritional stress. It is likely that much of the small average size of adults (and probably of older children) in Third World as compared to industrialized countries is the result of events in their lives which took place in the past. Although they may be eating less food as a result of being small, it does not follow that their size or any other aspect of their physical performance would be different if they had more food available to them after those early life experiences (although the quality of their lives might well have been). Second, the nature of that process of growth stunting has to do with the kinds of stress which involve the interactions between food and infectious disease, not necessarily with nutritional factors alone. This means that the common practice of referring to children who are small in height or weight relative to American or European standards as 'malnourished', and to the presence of such small children in a household or a population as an indication of inadequate food availability, is often wrong or even misleading. Smallness therefore is an indication that problems of stress either do or have existed. By itself, it tells us little about the kinds of problem that preceded it. Third, it seems reasonable in terms of the biology of the process that switching off the capacity of an individual to fully compensate for lost growth at quite an early age is an effective mechanism for a strategy of adaptation, whereby exposure to an adverse environment at the start of life results in a smaller and more economical adult.

More economical perhaps, but are there countervailing disadvantages? Is being small a bad thing in itself? Much time and effort have been expended in research trying to answer that question. Some of the findings are what we would expect. For example, that the maximum rate of doing work depends on the weight of muscle a person has and hence is broadly proportional to how big they are. But whether this is an advantage or not depends on the kind of work; other factors such as speed, dexterity or endurance can be important.

The heavy person is disadvantaged by needing more food even when resting than a lighter one, but, against that, someone who has survived a period of unemployment at the cost of losing a lot of weight may be unable to keep a job long enough to regain it.

That there are, and always have been, 'horses for courses', is clear from the range of sizes amongst relatively inbred tribal groups which still follow their traditional lives in different ecological settings. The achieved mean stature of such groups in Africa ranges between 144 cms for male pygmies and 147 cms for the bushmen of southern Kalahari to 176.5 cms for the Tutsi.[13] This is five times the range of heights amongst individuals in industrial populations. A study by Malcolm[14] of the growth of several tribes living in the highlands of New Guinea shows the mean stature of adult women as 12 cms shorter than the average European woman and intertribal differences of means of as much as 19 cms.

However, the much debated issue of whether small can be beautiful (or healthy) cannot be resolved easily. Some, for example Beaton,[12] incline towards the view that big is best on the grounds that, although moderate degrees of smallness are not known to be associated with any loss of functional capacity, they might nonetheless imply an unacceptable loss of potential for change, that is to say, a reduced ability of an individual to respond to new and possibly advantageous circumstances. This could be so – nobody knows. But loss of adaptive capacity (1) is an important cost only if such capacity is likely to be needed in future; (2) could as well be associated with non-adaptation as with adaptation; (3) above all, might be occasioned by any irreversible response – for example, by one that led to greater tallness, just as by a height-retarding response. Tallness closes some options, shortness others. Thus, while the jury may remain out for some time on the empirical effects of height and weight on health and fitness to actual or potential environments and lifestyles, there seems no reason to accept any a priori argument that 'taller' must mean 'more adaptable later' or otherwise 'better'.

In summary, there is at this time simply no agreement about a practical method for measuring the extent of undernutrition. It is likely that, in the near future, it will be suggested that a measure of 'thinness' based on some combination of weight and height could tell us whether or not a person is likely to have lost weight in the recent past.

However, the same confounding factors will operate and the controversy about the point at which adaptational changes give way to unacceptable damage will in all likelihood continue.

Is there anything more to be learned from past attempts? What, for example, is the meaning (if any) of the numbers in table 5.1? It is useful at this point to consider the hunger problem as having three elements.

First, were we able to agree on a method, it would obviously be desirable to estimate the numbers of people in whom the effects of hunger are manifested in some material way, that is, in whom symptoms of some overall disadvantage are currently present.

Having failed in that, we might at least ask about the numbers 'at risk' of experiencing hunger through failure of access to sufficient food. In practice, this would mean people whose ability to maintain control of their own food supply is in some way under constant or periodic threat. In fact, the methods used by FAO and the World Bank are based on a combination of available food supplies and income, that is, purchasing power. In other words, these are better thought of as estimates of the numbers of people who might only be able to purchase sufficient food to meet their estimated energy needs at the expense of forgoing other necessities. It could be argued that it is amongst that section of the population that individuals or households are to be found which, from time to time, fail to cope effectively with the combination of chronic poverty with additional chance misfortunes or illness and fall into the category of presently undernourished.

Obviously, the numbers 'at risk' will always be much larger than those presently or becoming undernourished at any one time – though by how much, we cannot say. It would not be wise to assume that the ratio of the numbers 'presently' to those 'at risk' is constant across different social, cultural or geographic divisions. It helps a little, however, to remember that the global estimates of 'at risk' of between one out of two and one in every five persons go along with global crude death rates (which will include deaths from starvation) of about 1 in 100.

One further stage would be to look at evidence for trends over time. Tables 5.4 and 5.5 have already shown evidence that both crude and first year mortality are on the decline. Although we cannot say how much, if any, of this is related to hunger, the decline in infant deaths is almost certainly an indication that the level of stress due to the nutrition–infection interaction is declining. Finally, we can refer to the FAO data on food supply per head of population, shown in table 5.7, to see that this is on the increase, remembering, of course, that this tells us only that there is more food available for people to buy, so long as they have the means to do so, on the countries' internal markets.

These regional and inter-country differences suggest that there is scope for equalizing the rates of improvement. However, and this may cause

Table 5.7 Food energy supply at country level in various regions

Region	*In 1965*	*In 1988*	*Rate of increase (% per year)*	*Population (millions)*
World	2390	2670	0.5	5210
Sub-Saharan Africa	2030	2010	0.0	480
East Asia	1940	2600	1.5	1520
South Asia	2060	2120	0.1	1130
S. America & Caribbean	2450	2740	0.5	420
Mid-income Countries	2122	2468	0.7	4052
Severely Indebted	2513	2805	0.5	554
High-income Countries	3080	3400	0.4	830

some surprise, I hope that the real significance of the better understanding we now have about the nature of the poverty–disease–food complex will be that there will be less rather than more advocacy of programmes which are specifically, and therefore perhaps narrowly, focused on bringing about nutritional improvements on the grounds that these are especially efficacious catalysts of further economic and social development.

The differences in rates of improvement in health indicators on average for the different regions are paralleled by differences in the rates of improvement in other conditions of life: educational attainment, especially of women, in the realm of general education, not just knowing about the properties of foods and techniques of child care (important though such knowledge may be); differences in the degree of equity, whether this relates to gender, to cash incomes or to access to open markets, to preventive health services, or to safe water.

If the concern is to reduce the differences in the underlying causes of the risk of hunger, then nutritional science gives us no easy escape from the conclusion that differences in poverty will have to be reduced. This is the basis for the view expressed earlier, that adopting a 'minimalist' view about the extent of overt hunger in no way involves the acceptance that doing so will result in more widespread attempts to offer cheap remedies – quite the reverse, in fact.

Famines Past, Present and Future

With this in mind, in the aftermath of the UN conference on the environment, it seems sensible to conclude with some comments about the longer-term prospects, not only of sustaining the current downward trends in the indicators of hunger, but also of the prospects for avoiding future recrudescence.

The discussion so far in this chapter has been about the question of the extent of chronic hunger. That is to say, the results of continuing situations of poverty and disempowerment. Even at this level, in order to make some sense of the relationship between the very high proportions of Third World populations seemingly at risk, and the relatively low and declining death rates, we found it helpful to think of life-threatening undernutrition as an acute and relatively infrequent phenomenon, generated by random or perhaps seasonal misfortunes, operating against a background of continuing risk factors. However, it is not too difficult to imagine a situation in which some kind of relatively sudden misfortune affects a large number of people or households at the same time or cumulatively over a short period.

This might happen because of one or a sequence of harvest failures, or because of a natural disaster such as flooding or earth movements which destroy food stocks and disrupt both food production and employment. We might further imagine that the scale of this is beyond the level at which existing networks of mutual support and self-help, through selling possessions, borrowing, calling in debts, temporary migration, and so on, are adequate to prevent starvation.

At a certain point in this rising tide of distress and failure to cope, the process becomes self-reinforcing. Because remaining food stocks are hoarded and not sold, prices begin to rise – except for livestock which, by contrast, can become almost valueless. Normal social obligations are ignored and public institutions for relief (if any existed) cease to function; large numbers of people abandon their land and homes and begin to move in search of relief; deaths from starvation begin to rise and this further damages both the cohesion and viability of households and then the functioning of public services and social organizations.

There are many variants of this process of the genesis of famine, depending on the normal pre-famine patterns of living, the extent to which people and social institutions have strong traditions of response based on past experience and, in more recent times, the extent to which external assistance is mobilized in time to prevent or ameliorate the effects of social disruption. My reasons for describing it are more related to the comment put into the mouth of the imaginary alien visitor at the beginning of the chapter. For a long time, people have held the view that if there were to be a Malthusian 'positive check' to population growth, it would be something which would creep up upon us in a rather gradual way. Perhaps a smooth rise in annual reports of deaths from starvation to a level which just balanced the rate of births. Perhaps also, many believe that this will simply seem like a return to a 'pre-developed' state for some less fortunate populations.

However, history and palaeoanthropology suggest that, in the past, mankind like many other large-bodied species has always made use of a range of mechanisms, physiological and/or behavioural in character, which provide a 'feedback' link whereby the current density of a population influences the subsequent reproductive performance of individual members. This results in populations which regulate themselves at levels which are always somewhat below the maximum that existing food supplies could sustain. Such self-regulated populations tend to vary in size more or less in parallel with food supplies, but do not seem to be limited by food in the short term; the observation that there are more animals where there is more food is commonplace, but examples of starvation are much rarer. This self-regulating strategy does not prevent the kind of famines which are the result of external or perhaps random processes, such as those described above.

However, it does prevent them being repeatedly and regularly caused by a population simply outgrowing the capacity of its own environment to provide a level of food energy which is sustainable in the long term. The reason why self-regulation of numbers is likely to be an inherited characteristic of large-bodied species is that those which lacked such mechanisms would be likely to damage their own ecological niche so severely that numbers could not regenerate in time to save them from extinction.

As for the prospect of avoiding a much more devastating and widespread Malthusian check, and as a change from looking at problems and solutions in the Third World, perhaps it would be as well to consider the prospects of sustaining our own food energy supply. Table 5.8, which is based on energy flow accounts calculated by Bayliss-Smith,[15] shows an analysis of the amounts of energy in the form of human labour, animal and machine power needed for food production at different stages in the development of agriculture. The values in the first row are for an example of a pre-industrial system, a tribe of people who cultivate food gardens in New Guinea in 1980. The values in the next are for Fyfield Manor Farm in Wiltshire for the year 1826, when it was visited by William Cobbett.[16] This row can also be thought of as representing the transitional production systems upon which a major part of the world's population still depends. The final row of values is derived from the energy budget for a mainly arable farm in the south of England in 1971. The increases in productivity mean that by 1971, one man was able to produce enough food for 200 people. However, whereas in 1826 higher productivity was achieved partly by using horses to supplement human effort, the really large increase since then has been achieved by using machines, which have now almost entirely replaced human and animal power. Productivity, however, has been bought at the cost of much lower efficiency of energy conversion. One unit of energy input in 1971 produced only two units of food energy, whereas in 1826 it produced 40.

Table 5.8 Labour and energy productivity of agriculture

	Labour productivity	*Energy input*			
	Days of food per work day	*Human*	*Animal*	*Machines*	*Ratio Output:input*
New Guinea 1980	1	100	0	0	14:1
Wiltshire 1826	7	77	21	2	40:1
South-east England 1971	200	0.2	0	99.8	2.1:1

Source: Gray, A. (ed.) (1993) *World Health and Disease*, Milton Keynes, Open University Press.

For the twentieth-century farm, we have to count as part of the inputs not only the fuel used by machines, but also the energy for manufacturing and transporting fertilizers, herbicides and insecticides. In 1971, each full-time agricultural worker in the UK was backed by non-agricultural energy inputs equivalent to 11.2 tons of oil fuel per year. Fyfield was an arable farm producing the cereal staple component of the national diet. However, some 35 per cent of our food energy comes from meat.

A high meat consumption has serious implications for energy use. The value of 2.1 units of food energy out for every 1 unit of input for a contemporary farm applies only to grains. Systems of animal production, many of which depend on specially grown feed crops, are even more inefficient, returning energy ratios of nearer 1:1.

Even these values only include processes as far as the farm gate. Modern supermarket provisioning involves complex systems of factory processing, packaging and storage. Continent-sized markets imply long-distance bulk transport, often followed by the use of personal car transport by individual purchasers. The energy costs of all of these are so variable as to be hard to represent meaningfully in a single value. However, one current estimate for the USA is that, whereas one farm worker can now produce the food needed by upwards of 1000 other people, every Kcal of food energy consumed requires on average a total expenditure of 9 Kcal (including the cost of an average of 2000 km of transport).

The food systems of industrial countries now account for nearly 20 per cent of their total energy use. Since this is mostly derived from coal and oil, it is of course solar energy which was trapped in plants millions of years ago. At first sight, this seems no different from the situation in 1826. This also involved trapping solar energy in fodder plants, feeding these to horses and using their muscle power to supplement human labour. The difference, however, is in the recycling of carbon. The same amount of carbon was simply exchanged back and forth between horses and plants, whereas carbon released from burning fossil fuels leaves a net increase in atmospheric carbon dioxide. In addition to carbon dioxide, the huge populations of ruminants (as many sheep as humans in the UK) excrete carbon in the form of methane, a gas which has an even greater 'greenhouse' effect than carbon dioxide. Food production in Third World countries also contributes to this: the green algae which live in rice paddies and contribute to their fertility are also a major source of atmospheric methane. In this way, the food production and distribution systems of both the industrial countries and the developing countries are now substantial contributors to the problem of global warming.

In 'Mass Extinctions', Norman Meyers[17] gives estimates of the size of the global population that could be equally provided with an average diet of the sort currently eaten in the UK without producing a continuous increase in the level of greenhouse gases and hence continued climatic change. This works out to be of the order of 2.5 billion. Barring a major catastrophe, the actual number alive in 2025 seems likely to reach nearer 8 billion, even if the most effective population policies are universally adopted.

This suggests that the kinds of questions which nutritional research should be addressing in respect of the future health of the industrialized countries should be not so much 'what is the composition of a diet which is optimal for health?' as 'what will be the health implications of a diet which is sustainable around the globe in the long run, assuming also an acceptable degree of equity?'.

NOTES

1 Rowntree, Benjamin Seebohm (1901) *Poverty: a study of town life*, London, Longmans, Green and Co.

2 Food and Agriculture Organization (1963) *Third World Food Survey*, Rome, FAO.

3 Food and Agriculture Organization (1977) *Fourth World Food Survey*, Rome, FAO.

4 Food and Agriculture Organization (1985) *Fifth World Food Survey*, Rome, FAO.

5 Alexandratos, N. (ed.) (1988) *World Agriculture: Toward 2000. An FAO Study*, New York, New York University Press.

6 Reutlinger, S. and Selowsky, S. (1976) *Malnutrition and Poverty: magnitude and policy options*, World Bank Staff Occasional Papers 23, Baltimore, Johns Hopkins University Press.

7 Reutlinger, S. and Alderman, H. (1980) *The Prevalence of Calorie Deficient Diets in Developing Countries*, World Bank Staff Working Paper 374, Washington, DC, The World Bank.
8 World Health Organization (1991) *Nutritional Strategies for Overcoming Malnutrition*, Executive Board Paper No. EB89/27, Geneva, WHO.
9 Lusk, G. (1928) *The Science of Nutrition*, Philadelphia, Saunders.
10 Keys, A., Brozek, J., Henschel, A., Mickelson, O. and Taylor, H. L. (1950) *The Biology of Human Starvation*, Minneapolis, University of Minnesota Press.
11 Benedict, F. G., Miles, W. R., Roth, P. and Smith, H. M. (1919) *Human Vitality and Efficiency under Prolonged Restricted Diet*, Washington, DC, Carnegie Press.
12 Beaton, G. H. (1989) 'Small but healthy? Are we asking the right question?', *Human Organization* 48 (1), 31–7.
13 Barnicot, N. A. (1964) 'Biological variation in modern populations', in G. A. Harrison, J. S. Weiner, J. M. Tanner and N. A. Barnicot (eds) *Human Biology*, Oxford, Clarendon Press, pp. 189–294.
14 Malcolm, L. A. (1974) 'Ecological factors relating to child growth and nutritional status', in Frank Falkner and J. M. Tanner (eds) *Human Growth Vol. 3: Neurobiology and Nutrition*, London, Baillière Tindall.
15 Bayliss-Smith, T. P. (1982) *The Ecology of Agricultural Systems*, Cambridge, Cambridge University Press.
16 Cobbett, William (1830) *Rural Rides*, Harmondsworth, Penguin English Library 1967, pp. 305–8.
17 Meyers, Norman (1992) 'Mass Extinctions', in *Global Catastrophes in Earth History*, Special Paper 247, Boulder, CO, Geological Society of America.

6

Eating and Being: What Food Means

Sidney Mintz

Asking what food means can bring forth answers that are in large measure either rhetorical or obvious. Like reproduction, eating unites all living things. The primal cry of the newborn human infant as it issues from the womb soon becomes a cry of hunger. And some of us, at least, depart life still eating, according to Dr Doran, an Englishman writing in the middle of the nineteenth century. 'Our sires used to make one curious use of sugar, undoubtedly,' Dr Doran tells us; 'namely, when they put it into the mouth of the dying, in order that the souls might pass away with less bitterness!' To eat, in other words, is to live.

Yet in the case of our species, the issue of meaning in food is real, for ours is the only species that wonders about what its food means – the only species that can even ask such questions. That there may be mysteries connected to the meaning of food is tied to our species' nature; such mysteries as there are, are mysteries that we ourselves have created.

In reflecting on what food and eating and their attendant mysteries mean, I shall restrict myself to a small number of themes, and there may be no harm in enumerating them at the outset. First, I wish to discuss the cultural, as opposed to biological, nature of human eating habits. Because food is essential to life, we may sometimes fail to take sufficient note of the socially learned character of our food habits.

Then I will look briefly at the history of food habits after the domestication of plants and animals, an achievement the importance of which was so great as to be nearly unimaginable. In dealing with domestication, however, my objective will be to put forward a rudimentary and hypothetical classification of food, one that might help us in comparing one cuisine with another. Though such comparisons tend to be made now in culinary or aesthetic terms, my purpose is rather to suggest that there were important parallels among different regions in the evolution of world diet in early times, after domestication.

I will introduce at that point a general assertion about changes in diet during the last five centuries or so, suggesting that a radical transformation has begun to occur, the long-term consequences of which are by no means clear. And I shall conclude by returning to the meaning of meaning in food, in order to offer a perspective which, while consistent with what is called structural anthropology, adverts to history in its approach to more thorough understanding.

If to eat is to live, then to live must be to eat. But what of Terence MacSwiney, the Lord Mayor of Cork? He won a special place for himself in the history books when, incarcerated under the Defence of the Realm Act in 1920, he embarked on a hunger strike in Brixton prison that lasted 74 days and ended in his death by coma. His act of protest excited international attention. If it can be said that MacSwiney lived on after his sacrifice, he did so by dying. And in that case, *not* to eat may be to 'live'. In any event, what became of MacSwiney's animal nature? His instinct of self-preservation? With such an instance in mind we might be tempted to conclude that, while there may be no mysteries in eating, there certainly may be some in not eating. But we would be wrong; there are mysteries in both.

Eating does unite all living things; but not all living things eat in the same manner, nor even with the same intentions. Our species stands alone, having resolutely created regimens of diet, and manners of eating, ludicrously remote from its animal nature. Clearly, not all members of our species eat the same things, any more than they speak the same language, wear the same clothes, or pray to the same god.

As a species that deals continuously in things that stand for something else, in 'representations', we have burdened the food we eat – and some would say all else in life, as well – with a backbreaking symbolic load. Food represents us; it sends our distinctive messages. Hence eating, like fasting, serves many purposes. 'I'm not hungry', can be a signal of great potency, as every anxious mother knows. Only of us human beings may it be said that when we are hungry, we may act sated; the capacity to dissimulate shows itself in eating behaviour as in all else. The same cannot be said of my cat, or your dog; when they act unconcerned about food, they've really had enough to eat. Here is a riddle known to nearly every young mother, at least in modern western society: why won't a baby eat what it needs – the way a cat or dog will?

But there is more than dissimulation to the mysteries of eating. In her pioneering studies of food and taboo, Mary Douglas, drawing upon Claude Lévi-Strauss, has called our attention to the ways that human groups categorize social reality conceptually. In Douglas' view, much of the mystery of food inheres in the structure of the abstract categories that society has created.[1] She has offered her readers a vision of tabooed foods as foods that straddle categories – the absence of scales, the presence of cloven hoofs – creatures with traits that will not fall into place, and so their flesh is deemed unclean. Her views have been challenged, but I think they have a convincing ring. Order is culturally inflected. Those substances which human beings are prepared to consume – which become, as it were, part of them – are subject to highly specific but often inexplicit rules of classification. Douglas' work aspires to uncover those rules.

The strong feelings of other cultures about certain foods, as revealed in their taboos, are not likely to surprise us, as long as we find the prohibited items repulsive. If, however, we are enthusiastic eaters of some of these tabooed foods ourselves, we may be somewhat hurt – or perhaps just condescending – when confronted with the visible disgust of others. The tabooing of pork by Moslems, like the tabooing of milk by many Asians, may appear to westerners as regrettable but excusable benightedness. But a sincere revulsion at the sight of a food we care about can seem to us unfeeling – indeed, insulting. We human beings are touchy about food: deeply affected by its colours, smells and the contexts of its consumption. We usually evince sturdy feelings of propriety about the cuisine we love.

That food can also excite strong positive feelings we all know and recognize. The tastes, smells, colours and textures of foods are enshrined among our earliest memories. Reawakened by association, they can take us back to our infancy: dependent, fragile, busily soaking up emotional and bodily nourishment in the arms or on the laps of those who made us human by teaching us to like the foods our culture deemed proper human food. Within this maturational process lies much of what foods can mean and, hence, much of their mystery.

People everywhere are certain that they not only know what is good for people to eat, but also that the way that they are human is somehow connected to their food habits. Why else do members of one culture so often find the food habits of another odd; or mildly unpleasant; or downright disgusting? Yet if we know nothing of the culture, we have no way of knowing what food its folk will consider delicious, and what repulsive. Because we humans eat so many different things, prepared in so many different ways, we learn to be prepared for surprises, even unpleasant surprises, when it comes to foreign food practices.

Eating habits, in other words, are not only acquired habits but also historically derived habits, uninscribed in our natures, except by early social learning. Though all peoples have ideas about what foods are good for them, in no culture do they eat everything. What is more, no people eats only what is thought to be good for them. Food taboos operate; and then, wittingly or no, they are broken. To be contrary, we might argue that taboos are made to be broken – not all of them at once, and for many people, never. But if there were no taboos, people would neither know what they ought not to eat, nor what to eat when they wanted to break a taboo.

Though all peoples have ideas about what is good for them, apparently many knowingly eat at least some things that may kill them – certain mushrooms, say; or the occasionally toxic blowfish the Japanese call *fugu*; or fish and shellfish from polluted waters, a North American weakness in these days of rising fish consumption and degraded environments and other delights.

But what people eat actually pales to near-insignificance alongside why people eat – and why they do not. Classical scholars tell us of those peoples who overate, and then made themselves vomit, simply for the pleasure of being able to eat more. Others starved themselves in order to get close to their gods. Yet others, as has already been noted in the matter of Mayor MacSwiney, starve themselves – to death, at times – to make a political point. How arresting is this aspect of our nature, that so fundamental a need of our physical selves may be stifled, at will, for one or more of a variety of other perceived goods.

In the USA there were those who formed picket lines and boycotted restaurants, to fight for the right to eat in the company of people they did not like. That was because breaking bread together – or, at any rate, next to each other – was correctly understood to be a powerful and nearly universal marker of equality. In certain highly stratified societies, such as India, the whole domain of food is deeply embedded in considerations of social, economic, political and religious identity, such that food and status are practically inseparable. No wonder that the eating behaviour of our species reminds us of no other animal – it is so unlike that of any other. Indeed, it might be said of this biological bedrock activity that human eating in culturally specific terms – and it always is culturally specific – is but barely connected to human biology at all.

This aspect of our behaviour has to do with the uniquely human capacity to create a symbolic world, and then both to call it reality and to treat it as real. But, as this discussion suggests, each such symbolic world – Aymara, Bemba, American – is a *different* symbolic world. It is precisely this staggering diversity of worlds of meaning, carried by members of one single species, that makes the human animal so special.

Though human beings have been seeking and successfully finding their food for perhaps three million years or more now, only in the last twelve millennia or so have they learned how to domesticate plants and animals, so that they could control the growth of their own food supply. Domestication means controlling the reproduction of some other living thing. It was not something invented just once, but many different times, and with different living things: rice, soybeans and pigs in Asia; potatoes, llamas and guinea pigs in the Andes; maize, tomatoes, chocolate, peppers and turkeys in Central America; millet, coffee and cats in Africa; olives and cabbage in Europe – all domesticated by nameless people, and bequeathed to all of us by a posterity that culture made possible. While we know the names and lives of Galileo and Copernicus, of Edison and Burbank and, for that matter, of the 'inventor' of the hula hoop, we know nothing of those many ingenious men and women, our ancestors, who invented domestication. In every case, the process from the feral species to that bred for specific characteristics desired by the domesticator was a lengthy and doubtless difficult one.

Domestication is the single greatest technical achievement in the human record, more important than the internal combustion engine or nuclear fission. Like these others, it was from the beginning a remarkable way to capture and control energy. But those other accomplishments were culminations of millennia of prior technical achievement – achievement made possible because of the benefits that once arose from domestication, and hard to imagine otherwise ever coming to be. Domestication was also and for very long a remarkably economical way to capture and conserve energy, when compared to the wasteful and dangerous uses we have made so far of fossil and nuclear fuels.

Coming very late in the whole human record, but very early from the point of view of forms of energy capture, domestication gave human beings an additional route to the understanding of time. Though the idea of time had doubtless been grasped in other ways, the control of the growth and reproduction of living matter provided a tremendous stimulus. The agricultural calendar gave time a new meaning; knowing when the rivers would rise or the first frost descend became even more important than before. Creating more exact measures of time – and, hence, mathematics – was in some measure an outcome of domestication. Learning to store food also took on added significance, part technical and engineering, and part mathematical. Genetics in the practical sense, of deliberately breeding plants and animals to enhance certain inheritable characteristics, was also an offshoot of domestication. From the point of view of the food quest, for many of the world's peoples it meant the eventual reduction or elimination of dependence upon caught and gathered food – though of course not completely. This saga, spread over millennia and over continents, remains central to our learning how to control our future.

In spite of the tremendous variety of plants and animals domesticated by humankind, over time it became clear that a relatively small number had become the subsistence mainstay of our species. So as not to complicate the story unduly, animals will not concern us here (though they certainly belong); plants will. Among the plants upon which our species gradually became dependent, there figured about a dozen grasses and perhaps an equal number of rhizomes or tubers. The grasses would include wheat, barley, oats, rye, maize, rice, buckwheat, quinoa and the millets. Not many more ever became important. The tubers would include manioc (cassava), yams, taro, sweet potatoes and potatoes. Again, few others ever became important. Around this baker's dozen of plants, most of the major societies in all of world history built their food supplies. Moreover, the increase in world population occurring in the very period when domestication was mastered makes it likely that the majority of human beings who have ever lived subsisted primarily on this rather small number of foods. Naturally, there was localization; rice, sweet potatoes and taro were important in Asia (though of course not only those); maize, potatoes, sweet potatoes and manioc were important in the New World; some millets and wheat were important in the Middle East; and so on.

But everywhere that one finds these grasses and rhizomes, plants rich in starch (the so-called 'complex carbohydrates'), one also finds one or more legumes to keep them company. The legumes or pulses are calorie- and protein-carrying plants: peas, beans, peanuts or groundnuts, chickpeas. They 'complement' the starchy foods, the complex carbohydrates. A Mexican tortilla complements red beans. In the Caribbean islands, red or black beans complement rice. In Asia, lentils (as dhal) and soybeans or soybean extracts, such as bean curd (fresh, dried, pressed or fermented) are important accompaniments to rice; in the Middle East, chickpeas commonly complement the wheat. Why a legume always accompanies a complex carbohydrate is not so easy to explain, though from the point of view of the human diet it is certainly a happy combination, particularly if the supply of animal protein (from fish, fowl or meat) is scanty.

Finally, everywhere that people eat one or more complex carbohydrates with one or more legumes, they also have flavours for their food. Calling them 'flavours' says too little; I shall try to explain what I mean by citing one of the most brilliant anthropologists of food who ever lived, Audrey Richards. In the following extract, Richards describes how an African agricultural people called the Bemba, whose principal food is a grain they cultivate, then turn into a gruel, eat this particular food:

> To the Bemba each meal, to be satisfactory, must be composed of two constituents: a thick porridge (*ubwali*) made of millet and the relish (*umunani*) of vegetables, meat or fish, which is eaten with it. . . . *Ubwali* is commonly translated by 'porridge' but this is misleading. The hot water and meal are mixed in proportion of 3 to 2 to make *ubwali* and this produces a solid mass of the consistency of plasticine and quite unlike what we know as porridge. *Ubwali* is eaten in hunks torn off in the hand, rolled into balls, dipped in relish, and bolted whole.
>
> Millet has already been described as the main constituent of Bemba diet, but it is difficult for the European, accustomed as he is to a large variety of foodstuffs, to realize fully what a 'staple crop' can mean to a primitive people. To the Bemba, millet porridge is not only necessary, but it is the only constituent of his diet which actually ranks as food. . . . I have watched natives eating the roasted grains off four or five maize cobs under my very eyes, only to hear them shouting to their fellows later, 'Alas, we are dying of hunger. We have not had a bite to eat all day'. . .

> The importance of millet porridge in native eyes is constantly reflected in traditional utterance and ritual. In proverb and folktale the *ubwali* stands for food itself. When discussing his kinship obligations, a native will say, 'How can a man refuse to help his mother's brother who has given him *ubwali* all these years?' or, 'Is he not her son? How should she refuse to make him *ubwali*?' . . .
>
> But the native, while he declares he cannot live without *ubwali*, is equally emphatic that he cannot eat porridge without a relish (*umunani*), usually in the form of a liquid stew. . . .
>
> The term *umunani* is applied to stews – meat, fish, caterpillars, locusts, ants, vegetables (wild and cultivated), mushrooms, etc. – prepared to eat with porridge. The functions of the relish are two: first to make the *ubwali* easier to swallow, and second to give it taste. . . . The Bemba himself explains that the sauce is not food. . . . Meat and vegetable stews are cooked with salt whenever possible, and there is no doubt that an additional function of the relish in native eyes is to give the porridge taste and to lessen the monotony of the diet.[2]

What Richards calls 'relish', I shall call fringe. Every cuisine has it, but perhaps it is particularly important in the diets of agricultural peoples who eat much complex carbohydrate. It 'helps the food go down'. It differs in many ways from the carbohydrate or basic starchy food, and some of those differences show up provocatively.

For the moment, perhaps the important thing is to see these three types of food as types, as categories, and not as particular foods. The starchy centre of the cuisine I call the 'core'; the flavour-giving foods I call 'fringe'; the protein-giving food I call 'legumes' (because that is what they are): core–fringe–legume. Together they form a pattern, which I shall call the CFLP. But before saying more about the CFLP, I want to distinguish more thoroughly among the categories, and illustrate them on one's plate. What is perhaps important to remember here is that I use the term 'pattern', meaning thereby that the particular food in each category is not so important as the category it exemplifies – that the items eaten stand in systematic relations to each other. Of course that is not at all the way the eaters think about them – they are interested in eating, not in some observer's devices for explaining things to himself. The particular foods are immensely important to the eater. Imagine convincing the Chinese to replace rice with black bread – or the Russians to replace black bread with rice! Eaters care about food, not about categories. They all have startlingly specific and explicit notions of what a good meal is, down to the precise textures of its ingredients. Like language, food is 'democratic'. Everybody speaks, but everybody knows and cherishes his own or her own particular language. Similarly, everybody has strong opinions on food, but those opinions are about specific foods, familiar foods, the 'right' foods. Yet for the picture of a pattern I am trying to develop here, the Chinese rice and the Russian black bread are to some extent interchangeable. That is because for the pattern to be perceived, it has to consist of 'slots' or categories, into which different things can be put in place of each other.

Let us imagine three different meals, to see how this might work. In the first, a broth or soup is made, using various fringe elements as well as one or more legumes. Into the soup on serving is ladled a substantial quantity of a pre-cooked starchy meal or flour, in order to make a kind of soupy stew or porridge. The dish is then eaten with a spoon. In the second cuisine, some kind of bread is baked or otherwise cooked from the flour of a cereal. Once it is baked, there is inserted into it – as if it were an envelope, a sheath or other container – a quantity of fringe foods and legumes. The resulting dish, rather like a large sandwich, can be eaten with the hands. In the third cuisine, a thick porridge or gruel is made from the rhizome of a starchy vegetative plant. It is then sprinkled with, or has stirred into it, additional foods, probably including some fringe elements; a legume may also be added, or it may be eaten separately instead. This flavoured gruel is then folded within an inedible leaf container, and in this form may be boiled, steamed or baked. It is unwrapped to be eaten. As will be grasped immediately, the appearance of these principal dishes varies greatly; but their composition, as illustrative of the tripartite principle I am suggesting, may be structurally similar. Examples of each of these major categories in specific cases may serve as illustrations.

The core, a 'starch', might be potatoes or maize, sweet potatoes or barley, yams or oats – that is, either a cereal or a rhizome. From such ingredients may be made a porridge, a bread or some sort of noodle – though that by no means exhausts the possibilities. The legume will vary similarly. In Latin America, it is commonly the red or black bean; in South-East Asia, the soybean or mung bean; in South-West Asia, the chickpea or lentil; and so on. As the tortilla is associated with Mexico, rice with South-East Asia and bread with the Middle East and Europe, so also *frijoles* are thought of as Mexican, bean curd as East Asian and *houmous* as South-West Asian. The fringe, because it may be thought of as being 'everything else', is rather harder to describe by example.

The difference between core and fringe seems always to be enshrined in the language itself, and in the way food is eaten. That a Chinese banquet has no rice is, among other things, a way of declaring that it is a banquet. That the proportion of fringe to core increases on ritual occasions is a way of saying it is a ritual occasion. That core without fringe would be tedious most of the time is understood; that fringe without core would be 'rich' – or even nauseating – is just as well understood. People seem often to be left wanting a 'little more' of some part of the fringe; but they do not normally imagine making a meal of the fringe. In other words, the formal distinctions which follow should not blind us to the fact that this difference is a living part of the way the world of food is organized for most people.

Perhaps the most striking difference between core and fringe is botanical: the core is always a complex carbohydrate, the fringe is probably never one. Another striking difference is likely to be texture: the core is always cooked, and always relatively soft and chewy (bread, rice, potatoes, tortillas, couscous, bulgur, boiled and mashed yams, hominy grits, taro or green bananas, manioc 'bread', buckwheat porridge, sorghum 'mealies', etc.). Texture is another customary difference: the core is almost always soft when contrasted to the fringe, if the fringe is solid; but the fringe may be mainly liquid in some cuisines. Cooking normally transforms the core into a softer substance with homogeneous taste and texture. The fringe may also be soft, or even liquid; but it may also be hard and chewy, or of any intermediate texture. Perhaps the most dramatic difference will be colour. The fringe is almost invariably more coloured than the core, and may even be quite violently coloured (red, golden, bright green; many-coloured, coloured with special dyes, black or dark purple or grey). The core is usually white or beige, or cream-coloured or some shade or shades of brown. But these features are merely introductions to the contrast. The real difference is taste: the fringe always has 'more taste' than the core; the core 'tastes better' with fringe; the fringe 'helps' one eat more core; the fringe by itself (like the core by itself, except under special ritual conditions) is less appetizing than the two combined. The ingredient(s) in the fringe may be from a cultivated or a wild source – to pick an example, wild dandelion leaves versus cultivated watercress. It may be plant (garlic) versus animal (cheese). It may be liquid (broth) versus solid (mushrooms).

The liquid–solid theme is an important basis for wide variation, and – as so often happens in matters of cross-culturally variable taste preferences – people may feel very strongly about the 'right amount' of liquid or solid in the fringe, complaining that the fringe is too wet, not wet enough, lumpy, not lumpy enough, and so on – messages with which many of us may be familiar, in one or another setting. The fringe may also be lukewarm or cold, rather than hot, while the core is hot – less commonly, the temperatures may be reversed. Usually there is a set of fringes, viewed to some extent in an order of preference that is generally accepted, with room for individual differences, but also partly subject to considerations of status, season, abundance or rarity, and so on. The preferred fringe (or fringes) may be salt (seaweed), sour (pickle), bitter (aubergine), sweet (fruit) or piquant (black pepper, cayenne, mustard, horseradish, ginger, and so on). They may be fresh (mint) or cooked (spinach), hot or cold, consisting of one ingredient or several; prepared by one mode of cooking (for example boiling) or more than one (for instance boiling plus broiling). The relation of a particular fringe food to the core may be more or less invariant (olive oil or Parmesan cheese to pasta, maple syrup to pancakes) or occasional (milk to cornmeal), and its culinary distance from the core – by which I mean the frequency, importance and meaning of its association – may also vary.

As we begin to examine the relationships between particular cores and particular fringes, it becomes clear – as I have sought to emphasize already – that what is constant is precisely the relation between core and fringe. The parallelism between core–fringe diets in widely different cultures, however, consists in something more: the central food, the major caloric source, is a 'starch'; the fringe consists of anything else, and usually many other things.

Obviously, a classification as simple as this cannot by any means serve to describe cuisines – that is not its purpose. But it can serve to make major cuisines comparable at a simple level. It has certain nutritional implications – but again, only of the simplest sort. It has historical implications, too, because it is based on the idea that certain parallels in cuisine emerged after the mastery of plant and animal husbandry. Implicit in the line of argument is the idea that these parallels became standardized to some extent, as complex political systems emerged, and territorial control was extended over large and environmentally different regions. Though this is not the place to advance these speculations, I would guess that such parallels also have to do with the emergence of *haute cuisine*. On the one hand, and for obvious reasons, culinary specialization could be expected to develop at the political centre – though, as Jack Goody has shown, that has not always been the case.[3] On the other hand, my own guess would be that much culinary specialization also developed at the peripheries of the political system, in reaction to the draining off of protein-rich foods by that same centre. Testing of such ideas must depend upon additional research.

To discuss meaning in the context of the cuisines of specific civilizations and cultures is beyond the purpose of this chapter. But anyone who has read of the mystical significance of maize in the case of American Indian peoples, of rice in the case of Asia, or of wheat in the case of the West, knows well how the imagery of particular foods can provide a governing idiom for life itself. Such predominance of particular plants or foods in the life of a society can be revealed in ritual, linguistic imagery, dress, coiffure and even literary texts. But here I wish to turn to quite another sort of meaning.

A few hundred years ago, the ancient and widespread core–fringe–legume pattern, highly diverse in detail but (I suspect) surprisingly similar from case to case in its organization and broad outlines, began to crumble. This happened first in Western Europe. Its deterioration came at roughly the same time as the Industrial Revolution. I think that this may not have been a coincidence. During the ensuing two centuries, the CFLP has decayed at ever-faster rates, over more and more of the earth's surface, hastened by large-scale migration, war and conquest, vastly improved technology of agriculture, animal husbandry, transportation and communication.

The main alternative foods, which have served to hasten the destruction of the ancient CFLP itself, fall into two principal categories. Both are typified by high caloric concentrations. Both stand in dramatic contrast to the starchy cores. Both can be consumed in varied fashion with the core foods. Indeed both, in one form or another, have certain very ancient associations with human appetite. At different times and in different ways, both have been affiliated culinarily with the core foods, but fitting in as rather minor parts of the fringe – prized, yet too scarce to be eaten often or in large quantities. At the same time, they did not become more important ingredients of world diet merely as arithmetically increasing fractions of the total caloric intake of world populations, making the core 'richer' or 'more nutritious'. Instead, they have gradually altered the nature of the core itself – its dietary, nutritive and ideological contribution, and its relations to other foods. What is more, it is probable that increases in worldwide consumption of these foods have implied fundamental changes in world energy use.

One of these two food categories consists of fats – animal fats such as lard and butter, and non-animal (seed, nut and vegetable) oils, such as corn (maize), palm, cottonseed, sesame, rapeseed, peanut (groundnut) and safflower oil. There are of course great differences between 'animal' and 'vegetable' fats, both in terms of their nutritive and health meanings for humans, and in terms of the nature and economy of their production. Yet I have put them together for the present argument. Whether the fat is animal or vegetable may be less important than its role in evolving mass diets. The most important modern example of these foods for our purposes is oleomargarine, a hydrogenated fat product now commonly made from vegetable oils.

The other such alternative food category consists of sugars – but so-called 'processed sugars', such as sucrose from cane, dextrose and (isomerized) fructose from maize, and so on, rather than the unprocessed sugars to be found in fruits and vegetables. The most important example for our purposes is cane sugar, made from the sugar cane, and beet sugar from the sugar beet: both of them undifferentiated sucrose. But here, too, from a different perspective, the particular source of the sugar matters rather less than the larger category of which all processed sugars are a part, so that there are some grounds for putting them together in terms of their function in the cuisine rather than segregating them in terms of their specific chemical, nutritive or molecular nature.

Both fats and sugars, including processed sugars, are 'natural', by which is meant here only that they can be extracted without alteration. Cane sugar (sucrose) is extracted from the sugar beet or sugar cane or sugar palm, just as cottonseed oil is extracted from cottonseed, palm oil from the oil palm, and so on. None need have any other ingredient added to it. (The extraction and processing of animal fats, however, does raise special technical problems, which cannot be addressed here.)

Together, fats and sugars (both in the ways that they are made and in the ways that they are conceived and combined) have modified our human relationship to nature, while playing a special role in the remaking of the food habits of the entire world. That remaking, however, has been uneven and, as noted earlier, it happened first in the west, particularly in Western Europe. It happened next in the European (or 'white') colonies or erstwhile colonies – such as the United States, Canada, Australia, Argentina, South Africa, and so on. It has now begun to happen in much of the world at large, including the old colonial areas of the west (such as Africa, the Caribbean and South-East Asia), and in what once was called the socialist world. This massive change, whereby sugars and fats have gradually begun to replace the complex carbohydrates of the core, and thereby to erode the structure of the meal itself, I refer to as the 'second revolution'. If the first revolution was domestication, perfected a few thousand years ago, then the second revolution is now much less than five centuries old.

It seems to me that the way CFLP eaters become big consumers of fats and sugars is not via some single, undifferentiated vector, but comprises different ongoing processes, some still poorly understood, that I have grouped together under the term 'second revolution'. Our understanding of how food habits change, both historically and at the present time, remains incomplete. Hardly anywhere, apparently, is the value of a change from one way of eating to another carefully weighed or questioned by consumers, who often seem to be 'thinking about something else' besides eating and drinking, when they are learning to consume a new product. A good illustration of a modern new food that has wrought great changes in a short time, almost unnoticed, is the so-called 'soft drink', usually a carbonated, heavily sweetened, flavoured drink served cold. A trivial product consumed by a tiny minority of the world's population 75 years ago, the soft drink is now almost as widely diffused as salt. In the US, more soft drinks are consumed than water. This beverage continues to spread widely, and has been taken up by both the Russians and the Chinese, particularly in the popular western 'cola drink' forms, without hardly so much as a ripple of doubt. Changes of this kind continue to occur often without being understood and, even less, studied, though their long-term cumulative impact on traditional food habits may be considerable.

It is by describing the second revolution, as I call it here, that I return to the matter of meaning. In my book, *Sweetness and Power*, written in 1985, I dealt with increases in the consumption of sugar in the United Kingdom in the period *c.*1650–1900, especially in association with the hot stimulant beverages. I argued that there was no single convincing reason why Britons and their neighbours had so enthusiastically taken up the consumption of tea and like stimulants. But poor nutrition, a cool and rainy climate and the compelling rhythm of the industrial workday may have combined to make this change a highly likely one, when sugar and tea became known and affordable.[4]

In the course of my argument, I asked what might be said about meaning in this connection, particularly in view of the transformation of these once rare and costly exotica, tea and sugar, into everyday proletarian necessities. In a case of this kind, it seemed to me not quite enough to talk about the structure of cuisine, or the symbolic significance of the contrasts within it, in explaining what foods mean. I would want to know how long people had been eating particular foods, where those foods came from, how expensive they were, and how different groups and classes felt and thought about them, before attempting to decide what they meant. When analyses of meaning in a case of this sort proceed without reference to such questions, then meaning must be defined as embodied in the foods themselves – the arrangement of foods betokens a symbolic structure, a timeless representation that conceals meaning within itself. Of course there is a question about what we take 'meaning' to mean – within what limits of space or time we choose to define what things mean. But one notices the way British food habits changed – the replacement of home baking with shop-bought breads, of home-brewed ale with tea, of butter with jam, and so on. One notices, too, how food habits percolate downward to some extent, from the privileged classes to the labouring classes, and how working people themselves transform eating patterns to fit their own needs. Under these circumstances, an analysis that does not take into account prices, advertising, the advice of doctors and other professionals, or the social conditions under which a new food is added, including the intentions of producers, retailers and the state, must omit certain kinds of meaning. I wanted to know where these new foods came from, why they succeeded, who benefited from their production and sale, how their prices had changed. The answers to such questions were clearly quite different from those concerned with the internal symbolic structure of the meal, where meaning can be understood as the underlying conceptual vision of those doing the eating. For my purposes, structural analyses of the meal based on contrasts between hot and cold, wet and dry, solid and liquid, revealing and insightful as they are, do not tell me all that I want to know. The meanings imparted to these new foods by those who consumed them were real enough. I called them 'inside meaning' in *Sweetness and Power*. But I wondered about a whole different assemblage of meanings, which I referred to as 'outside meaning'.

The terms 'inside meaning' and 'outside meaning' represent a rather crude distinction between historical and non-historical approaches to what is meant by 'meaning' in the study of cultural activities such as eating. In effect, the cultural materials people employ in creating systems or symbols – foods are a suitable example of such materials – are not givens, but are the precipitate of economic, social and political processes. Sugar, in the case which interested me, was a relatively new substance for the British people, one which travelled downward in the class system from royalty to the people, meanwhile taking on all kinds of particular symbolic meaning. But in my view, the availability of sugar, the medical arguments made in its defence, the interests of the planters, the slave traders and the merchants, the taxing power of the state, all enter into a discussion of what sugar meant to those who consumed it. I thought it not enough to decode the meaning of the meal; I needed to decode the codifiers.

In this discourse on the meaning of eating, I have quite deliberately sought to consider some different ways to think about what eating means, rather than dealing in greater detail with one such meaning. The study of food and eating is still not well understood, at least in the social sciences. That so vital an activity should remain enigmatic ought not to discourage us; think how long, and with what limited success, we have wondered about the significance of love and loving. One can merely hope that, in the case of food and eating, we have greater chances of eventual success.

NOTES

1 Douglas, Mary (1966) *Purity and Danger*, London, Routledge & Kegan Paul.
2 Richards, Audrey (1939) *Land, Labour and Diet in Northern Rhodesia*, London, Oxford University Press.
3 Goody, Jack (1982) *Cooking, Cuisine and Class*, Cambridge, Cambridge University Press.
4 Mintz, Sidney W. (1985) *Sweetness and Power*, New York, Viking Penguin.

FURTHER READING

Salaman, Redcliffe (1949) *The History and Social Influence of the Potato*, Cambridge, Cambridge University Press.

Simoons, Frederick (1967) *Eat Not This Flesh*, Madison, University of Wisconsin Press.

Weismantel, Mary (1988) *Food, Gender and Poverty in the Ecuadorian Andes*, Philadelphia, University of Pennsylvania Press.

7

Food Symbolism, Gender Power and the Family

Ann Whitehead

Some Representations of Gender and Food

There are very many terrains on which the relation between food and gender can be discussed. There is of course an immediate practical, physical or economic level. For example, food production, food provision and food preparation are everywhere activities marked by sexual or, more properly, gender divisions of labour. These may be more or less rigid and more or less subject to social valuation and sanction. Men and women usually consume unequal amounts of food, and there is evidence that, in some places, the sexes suffer and survive modern-day hunger and malnutrition differently. A material dimension to the link between food and gender is illustrated in various ways by three treatments in film.

First, let us look at *Saturday Night and Sunday Morning*, based on Alan Sillitoe's novel which was set and made in 1950s Nottingham and noted for its social realism.[1] Here the hero, Arthur, is seen first in the factory, then coming home, and finally being served at the table by his Mam, while his Dad watches television. Arthur represents rebellious youth out for a good time. He is antagonistic to the old ways of the working-class family, community and factory which are remorselessly depicted in visual image, in the music and in the dialogue of the film. Eating in the home is depicted as segregated in time and space, with neither men and women, nor in this case older and younger, eating together. The timing of the hot evening meal, it seems, is related to homecoming from work. Cooking and serving the meal is the work of the mother/wife and is presented in a direct exchange for part of the son's wage. There is a suggestion too that the mother is more indulgent to her son than to her husband.

A second set of representations of the material aspect of the link between gender and food is found in a television programme made at the height of the African famines of the mid- to late 1980s.[2] Here the important roles of women in farming, and also in providing domestic food, in conditions where most of the activities needed to transform the food from raw harvest to palatable meals are undertaken by a woman in the home, with little in the way of technology, are graphically portrayed. Women are also shown caring for children who are dying of starvation.

The third cinematic example is from an ethnographic film about a community in the forests of Brazil.[3] This film takes the relations between the sexes as its main theme. It is argued that the economic interdependence of the sexes is expressed in rituals of sexual antagonism. Gender hostility and aggression has to be continually re-enacted in rituals which punctuate the Mehanicu year. The film concentrates on the rituals placating the spirits on which food abundance and human welfare depend, one of which involves the myth of the origin of the piqui fruit, an important food staple for the Mehanicu, a myth which is closely linked to women and their sexual activity.

The third example shows that, in addition to its material significance, food carries complex cultural meanings. Within any culture no item of food is ideologically innocent. Think of muesli and beefburgers, smoked salmon and prawn cocktail, chocolate eclairs and steamed jam pudding. A European reader will, however, not be able to contextualize another cultural repertoire with which I am familiar – shall we say fufu and light soup, kulikuli, TZ, and Milo – all of which can be socially placed by Northern Ghanaians. The cultural meanings carried by specific items of food, and by practices around food, usually relate to class and ethnicity, to age, and to gender, sex and sexuality.

For example, although at the immediate level the cinematic example about famine seems to lack this symbolic dimension, the choice of women and children to represent Third World vulnerability to famine and hunger is also not 'ideologically innocent'. We get a dual message, which is more powerful than one in which men are shown starving.

For a second example, in another episode in *Saturday Night and Sunday Morning*, Arthur is served a breakfast by his married woman lover, after spending the night with her. She does not eat or sit down with him, and as he is finishing, her husband and young son arrive back at the house. Arthur has to creep out, after wiping his plate with a piece of bread. Here Arthur's meal is used to symbolize his usurpation of the marriage bed. In another part of the film, being invited home to tea is part of the appraisal that Arthur has to undergo in his courtship of his other girlfriend, this time young and unmarried. Her mother pronounces him a bit rough, but this is all part of his attraction for the girl.

The scene has then been set. In this chapter, both the material and the symbolic dimensions to the link between gender and food will be explored. I shall concentrate on the allocation of food within the family.

Rituals of Allocation

Food allocation within the family or any other regular eating group is usually sufficiently conventional in form as to amount to a ritual, or set of rituals. Let me give two examples. The first is from the Ecuadorian Andes, from a study of a community called Zumbagua by Mary Weismantel.[4] In her introduction, she comments:

> In Zumbaguan minds the image of the hearth is intrinsically associated with that of the woman as mother, wife, daughter, daughter-in-law. The whole conceptual framework that I have called cuisine is considered to be the exclusive possession of the female sex; although men are perfectly competent cooks, they consider their cooking to be an ad hoc improvisation attempted without the benefit of women's knowledge.

The allocation of food during a harvest meal is described in the following terms:

> Zumbagua houses lack tables, so everyone eats scattered around the room on benches or on the floor, eating soup out of tin bowls and tossing bones to the dogs. Despite the apparent haphazardness, a strict hierarchy is observed in the seating arrangements. Tiny chairs or low seats are offered to the most honoured diners, usually the senior male(s). Then according to a flexible series of social criteria that puts old before young, male before female, and guest before host, others are seated on still lower seats or on cloths or straw spread on the floor. As a general rule, men sit above the ground while women sit on it. . . .
>
> The order in which people are served is another indication of social status. Decisions regarding this order belong to the woman doing the serving from the (cooking pot) normally the senior woman of the house.

The women at the cooking pot can also express the difference in status among the eaters, and her own sense of their personal esteem, by the kinds of bowls and spoons they are given. Here there is no 'matching dinner service', but a 'wide discrepancy in size, shape, design and materials' from which bowls and spoons are made. This variety is anything but haphazard and is instead used to 'emphasise the social inequality of those who eat together', with the most important getting the largest, best decorated and most valued bowls and spoons.

Equally important is the food itself. A main meal consists of potatoes or barley and a soup. But the Zumbaguan soup is not an amorphous dish, ladled so that the consumer takes 'potluck'.

> Each bowl of soup is carefully constructed, meats, vegetables and broth being apportioned with a specific consumer in mind. . . .

> This act of composing each bowl of soup is an acknowledged stage in making a meal. There is nothing furtive about a woman's fishing about in the soup pot, looking for more pieces of cabbage to add to a serving, or putting some back if she gave someone too much. Selecting potatoes, or poking through the meat dish to find just the right piece, is done with a flourish: a woman thus displays her skill in assembling a filling, aesthetically pleasing, and socially appropriate serving.

Although this is a description of a meal where guests are present, 'all the ritual of the meal is still present in even the most intimate and casual of family meals' and 'it is still conceived of as a gift, from parents to children, from woman to man'.

There is obviously a great deal of practical and social skill involved in the woman's allocation from the cooking pot, and it is not surprising therefore that a young married couple, although they have their own rooms, will continue to eat and cook with parents long into their married life. It may be up to ten years after they have married before they establish their own kitchens.

In the second example, Britain, no single description would be appropriate, given the enormous variation in the economic and sub-cultural circumstances in British families. Indeed, popular reports of the growth of grazing (eating without sitting down, often on the street), of meals sitting in front of the television, of fast food and take-away, suggest that shared and family-provided meals may be in serious decline.

However, a recent full study in York[5] suggests that, for families with dependent children, there remains a strongly articulated notion of the place of meals in family life. There was a remarkably common cross-class set of elements in values and practices. Most women had a clear notion of what was a proper meal, and held the view that good family life was signalled by such meals. The cooked meal on Sunday was the proper meal, par excellence, and was a main weekly occasion for cooking and eating.

Although the study does not give ethnographic descriptions of observed meals, it is clear that meals in these families too are ritual occasions, with allocation as one element in the ritual.

One stereotype of allocation is shown in *Saturday Night and Sunday Morning*. The son of the family is served at the table, set in a careful way, by his mother, who does not sit down, or appear to eat herself. His father was given a post-meal cup of tea, as he sat watching TV.

In one-third of the families studied in York, husbands ate separately during the week from the rest of the family. The authors of this study also record inequality in the foods eaten by men and women. Red meat, better meat, cakes, cream and puddings go disproportionately to the men. We can observe that eating separately, justified in terms of the exigencies of man's working hours, easily facilitates this kind of inequality. It provides the opportunity for the husband/father to receive the better cuts of meat, the rich pudding, and the cooked dinners which constitute 'proper meals'. The wife/mother may have eaten a more 'snack-like' meal with her children earlier.

In the UK in general, a prime occasion for rituals of allocation occurs at what for virtually all families remains the main meal of the week – the Sunday dinner/lunch/supper. There are families where carving is the man's task at this meal, and this may, or may not, be associated with his control over portions – who gets what especially of the central meal element, or whatever is defined as the choicest, most expensive, or most nutritious. In some households, no doubt strict equality is the norm, but there is plenty of evidence that different kinds of meat, or other food, are either thought more suitable for those of different sex and ages, or are served unequally to them. Conventionally, for example, the red meat of the legs and thighs of chicken and turkey usually go to men, and the white meat for children and women.

However, it is common for the distribution of the main Sunday meal food to be done by the woman. It is more likely then for the meat to be cut up by the woman in the kitchen than carved at the table. Although the distribution may be then done by individuals helping themselves, from all food served centrally on the table, it is more common for it to be served by the woman from the dishes on the table, which gives her an opportunity to control who has what.

In yet other families the food may well be 'plated' before serving – that is, all the elements of the meal placed on individual plates meant for particular members of the household, and then served on to the table. This provides the greatest opportunity for female control. I was brought up in a three-generational family, during post-war rationing, when food was scarce. In my early childhood (though this changed later), the tensest moment of our Sunday dinner was the last few minutes when all the various elements of the meal had to be simultaneously hot and ready, and were then served onto the plates for each family member ('that's your father's', 'that's Pop's', etc.).

In my household, the plates were arranged by my mother, but my grandmother always came to check the servings before we two daughters took them to the table. She could never resist moving a few pieces of meat or vegetable about from plate to plate so that each family member had what she regarded as their due. My memory was of a strict hierarchy of allocation, in which larger size and better quality went to my grandfather and father. In this allocation, my mother reserved the poorly shaped, or the worst cooked, or less succulent pieces for herself.

Example after example, across the world, from Europe, from India, or from sub Saharan Africa, can be found to show that food allocation within the household is marked by more or less degrees of formality and convention. Within these conventions, it is rarely the case that the allocation of food is equal.

Commensality, eating together, marks social division as frequently as it demonstrates social solidarity. Particular kinship or family statuses such as being a daughter-in-law, senior wife or head of household, being old, being young, being adopted, being last born or first born, being boy or girl, can all be the opportunity for special treatment, good or bad, in the patterns and rituals of family food allocation.

My concern here is with the gender dimension to these patterns of allocation, and moreover, with the fairly widespread finding that men, or at least some men, are often deferred to in food-serving rituals, and that they may get more, or better, food. This is particularly true of 'senior men' – however seniority is culturally defined.

We should note two caveats at the outset. Of course in the UK, at formal dinners at home and outside, 'ladies first' is the rule. Here I am looking at family meal situations where there is not a lot of evidence that this convention operates. Secondly, one other dimension in these patterns which is taken for granted is that of age. An exactly parallel analysis to the one I am about to make for gender could also be made for age, but that would be the subject of another study.

If we can confine discussion to gender, the first obvious question is whether there is any material or physiological significance to these widespread findings. In the British case, quite a strong argument can be made that, in conditions of overall food adequacy, the priority given to male food preferences and to male appetites is now detrimental, given the apparent link between diet and the diseases of affluence (see chapters 3 and 4 in this volume). All that red meat, cream and those starchy puddings – more likely to kill than to preserve!

Globally, however, there are more social situations where the quantity and quality of food is undersupplied than oversupplied. This raises the substantial question: in conditions where there is not enough food, or not enough food of the right kinds, are there any physiological implications of the fact that food-serving etiquettes tend to give men primacy? Or, to put it another way, do family food allocation patterns lead to women's hunger?

Nutritional Adequacy and Family Food Allocation Patterns

It is immediately necessary to admit that, in asking this question, we are confronted with a methodological minefield. It is one thing to observe the kinds of rituals of allocation just described, and quite another to measure real food intakes, from all sources, for a whole 'average' day, for each family member and to determine their nutritional equity. For that evaluation raises the issue of food needs.[6] If food intakes were equal and identical, this would not necessarily be a situation of equity if food needs differ, which they do. In any case, recommended intakes do not deal with individual variations, such as those due to differences in physique, physiological state and energy expenditure. These could make any particular woman's nutrient needs greater than those of her male partner.

All this in situations where we cannot 'experiment' by deliberately engineering physiological or energy-expenditure differences in populations, and where variables often operate through feedbacks. Infectious disease produces loss of appetite and increases need for energy. There is, moreover, evidence that there are differences in the extent to which men and women can adapt physiologically to insufficient food. Further interpretive difficulties arise because any analysis of nutritional equity within households ought to be disaggregated at the community level in order to take into account the economic differences between them which affect aggregate household nutrients availability. The latter will also be affected by the point in the seasonal agricultural cycle at which surveys are done.

It is hardly surprising, then, that the findings on the link between patterns of food allocation and women's nutritional welfare are often difficult to interpret. The area where this debate has been examined most carefully is in India and Bangladesh.

Most South Asian cultures also have a complex set of beliefs about food, whose type and serving symbolize aspects of social relations. The centrality of these beliefs to Hindus is most familiar to us in the way in which food figures in pollution beliefs in relation to caste boundaries and caste behaviour. Eating together is a mark of sameness but there are gender dimensions to Hindu practices too. For example, it is generally regarded as improper for men to eat in the immediate company of women. Women eat after their husbands, and last. In some areas some 'prestigious' foods are never eaten by women, while the word 'leftovers' may be used for women's food. These 'leftovers' are the portions of food left when men have been served, rather than the leavings on men's plates. However, the word 'leftovers' graphically conveys differences in the kinds of claims that husbands and wives are making on the family food.

In South Asia, this complex of food behaviour exists side by side with considerable sex differences in mortality and morbidity. In many areas, and for many age groups, more females die than males, with the result that South Asia has an excess of males over females. This male sex ratio is noteworthy because it is in contrast to most other parts of the world, where females tend to predominate. Until recently the maleness of the population was tending to increase.

This is sufficiently striking to have produced a widespread academic and policy debate about its causes. One strand of enquiry has been whether there is any link with the nutritional adequacy of female diets in India and Bangladesh. The question is: are female family members discriminated against so that proportionally less of their nutritional needs are met, through these family allocation practices?

The household level studies which examine individual male and female food intakes have recently been exhaustively examined by Barbara Harriss. She finds that, although 'there is evidence of discrimination in feeding practices and nutrient allocation within the family in South Asia . . . it is rarely of a dramatic nature'. Gender-based nutrients discrimination against women is confined to the north and not always evident there. She finds also that the groups discriminated against in terms of calories are more often than not young children and the elderly, rather than adult women, although the allocation to women who are pregnant and lactating is probably not 'fair'.[7]

In other words, there is no confirmed general finding that adult women in South Asia are nutritionally disadvantaged more than men, despite family food practices in which they are treated as inferior. Barbara Harriss points out that these findings are counterintuitive, given the excess of female mortality in many age groups. Indeed, her analysis of the research findings has aroused dismay in some quarters and incredulity in others. Nevertheless, as she points out, there are a large number of other factors which affect female well-being, and which could lead to excess mortality – not least of these are women's work burdens, in both productive and reproductive spheres, and also the care and health treatment such women receive. What is interesting in her findings are the implications for how we interpret the patterns of food allocation with which this chapter began. They suggest that for gender, as well as for other statuses, family food allocation rituals may be about something other than physical access to nutrients. They should not be interpreted simply as ways in which family members get access to food resources, either equally or unequally, but rather as statements about something else. The remainder of this discussion will be concerned with what this 'something else' might be.

Food Symbolism in the British Family

To answer this question, I want to look more carefully at the place of meals in family life in the UK, using the study mentioned earlier in York,[8] and research done in South Wales by Anne Murcott.[9] Both studies found that women and men are attached to the idea of a 'proper meal'. The proper meal is a cooked dinner of meat (or fish), potatoes and vegetables, and is one which the family members sit down together to eat. The authors of both studies stress the central role of this cooked dinner in peoples' ideals of family life. It comes to stand for normal living as well as symbolizing, for the wife/mother/housewife, her abilities and competence and that 'all's right in the world'. Women who cannot provide proper meals, especially Sunday dinner – for example if they are on income support – feel that this symbolizes the way in which poverty affects the capacity to be a family. The studies also report the prodigious and often touching efforts made by men who have become the sole carers for their children to keep these routines going: 'I cooked Sunday dinner every week after my wife left', reports one father.

Both studies bring out how, to a striking extent, the organization and character of family meals is dominated by men's needs and preferences. The researchers argue:

> children learn of their father's superior authority along with the food they eat. Their choice is limited and subordinated to his preferences, at the main meal of the day, while at other meals, where he is more often absent, they may have more choice.[10]

In British families, the preference given to the man's food tastes, and the larger quantity and superior quality of adult men's food, is often justified in terms of physiological need – perhaps on the basis of their size or energy requirements. Arguably, this is a rationalization in at least two senses. First, this notion of need appears to be used whether or not there is evidence of any objectively greater need (smaller men or older, less active men still have 'masculine food needs'). Second, the needs being signalled, far from being material, are essentially symbolic. These family food practices serve to signal that the man/husband/father stands at the apex of the hierarchy of status within the family.

Cross-culturally, the extent to which this hierarchy is present varies enormously. But so too does the extent to which the ways in which women serve food contain elements of servitude and deference. I suspect this ambiguity in service, serving and servitude arouses quite strong feelings for some women when they cook and provide meals. A particular aspect of femininity is mobilized. This may be one of the differences when men cook, not just occasionally, but more or less all the time. In the absence of any research in this area, my speculation would be that while such men may feel they are caring and nurturing, they do not feel they are serving.

Both of the British studies also bring out the strong elements of affection and love with which food is offered by wives/mothers to the family. Women in all the studies report pleasure at feeding their children, and often pleasure at getting special food for the husband, or getting the proper meals 'right'. In this sense, the meals cooked and served by the wife/mother are a gift. But this giving is tarnished by many other meanings. One of them has already been dwelt upon – the element of servitude that may be present in the rituals of serving. In North Indian families, newly married daughters-in-law show enormous deference to male family members when they serve them food, and their own food is of poor quality, eaten furtively. It might be said that their family position is little better than a servant.

Returning to the British studies, it was found that many women express bondage, in other ways, in the sense that cooking, as with many other aspects of housework, is not done from choice, and is hard, relentless work. For women, meals as a gift cannot be separated from this work. But the giving element is also tarnished because, if men are constructed as having needs which must be met, women are constructed as self-denying. In earlier work I have described how in many cultures motherhood is constructed as being about altruism – putting the needs of others first.[11] This altruism is symbolized in the overt way in which food is allocated and meals are organized in British families.

In important ways, then, children learn more than male authority and table manners along with the proper dinner. They learn about the gendered selves: personhood is constructed and reproduced in family meals. Family food practices express a great deal about gender power. These constructions both structure the way men and women feel, and are not the full story about how they feel. The self-denying mother may feel greedy about her needs and the father may feel deeply that he would prefer his children to be well fed in preference to himself. At this level we begin to understand eating disorders and their relation to femininity, and some of the problems of masculinity.

In the UK, cooking is gendered in at least one other way. In her research on South Wales families, Anne Murcott found not only that a proper cooked dinner is the most valued meal, but also that the term 'cooking' is used to refer to a restricted set of meanings in meal preparation.

> 'She does not bother to cook at all. He is quite happy to have cold meat with a few boiled potatoes.'

> 'I often buy things like that – little individual pies for the nights for one reason or another when I don't feel like cooking.'

Men, as husbands and fathers, might quite often be responsible for meal preparation – as, for example, in 'getting breakfast'. But using the toaster and assembling cereal and milk are not dignified by the term 'cooking'. I find this very suggestive. It parallels the Ecuadorean men's view that their cooking or food preparation is 'ad hoc'. There, how to prepare full meals – using the right set of semiotically balanced items which are also nutritionally good, and hot, and timely, and which, moreover, are part of a set of such meals so that, during the week, there is variety, freshness, good nutrition and probably also thrift – this is all women's knowledge alone. It is this which is 'cooking'. In other words, cooking knowledge and cooking are constructed as gendered, even though both sexes prepare meals.

In the same way that the proper dinner symbolizes ideas of family life, 'cooking' could be interpreted as symbolizing the interdependence of husband and wife. By making cooking a female pursuit, a man cannot manage on his own. He may make meals, but he cannot cook – that is, provide the proper dinners which are at the heart of the family's life.

So, the idea of cooking as esoteric female knowledge carries the meaning of male dependence within marriage. Marital dependence is, of course, not one-sided. There are parallel female dependences symbolized in the way in which husbands 'and wives' incomes are treated in family budgets, in gendered inheritance rights . . . but those are other stories.[12]

This constructed, necessary interdependence, through ideas about cooking, reminds us of the theme of the Mehanicu film: the acute interdependence of the sexes in subsistence. It was argued that this kind of interdependence engendered anxiety, and even hostility and aggression, between the sexes. The aggression at the necessary interdependence of the sexes is a matter of shared culture. In the UK, there is less cultural stress on public rituals of hostility and aggression between the sexes. The acceptance of dependence and interdependence in marriage, which is always a complex emotional and economic matter, is mainly played out at the personal level. But it is not altogether surprising to find in the British studies that there is evidence that food, cooking and meals can be the focus of conflict, and of rage, in British families.

Domestic Violence: What's This Muck?

The darkest side of these complex linkages between domestic gender relations, the symbolism of cooking, ideas of femininity and masculinity, and gender power, is to be found in the link between food and the triggering of domestic violence.

Ellis, reviewing such research as exists for the UK, suggests that trouble between husbands and wives leading to wife assault often centres on meals. She reproduces a number of accounts from wives who have taken refuge from violent husbands:

> 'He does not like waiting for his meals, so if his supper is not being walked on to the table as he walks in the door – there is trouble.'

> 'A month ago he threw scalding water over me, leaving a scar on my right arm, all because I gave him a pie with potatoes and vegetables for his dinner, instead of fresh meat.'[13]

But this kind of behaviour is not confined to the homes of wife batterers. Kerr and Charles in York report the following from an interview with a husband and wife:

> The husband began by saying:
>
> 'There was once where you made something I didn't like – I remember that.'
> Wife: 'Oh yes, I forgot about that.'
> Husband: 'Yeah – But apart from a broken plate and a rather dirty wall there was no other damage.'
> Wife: 'I forgot about that altogether.'
> Husband: 'Yeah, I threw it at you didn't I? Do you remember?'
> [Did you?]
> Husband: 'Yeah. Oh dear me, I think I said something like, "Shove that fucking muck" – Oh, sorry the tape's on isn't it? I don't want to be rude. That was when we'd just got married wasn't it and you thought that was an acceptable standard of nourishment.'
> Wife: 'I thought it was nice, it tasted nice.'
> [That was right at the beginning of your marriage?]
> Husband: 'That's right, yeah. She's never given me any of that rubbish again so that's all right.'[14]

When I have begun to discuss this link between meals and domestic violence with other anthropologists, most of them have said that they too know situations where domestic violence is associated with husband's demands that their wives provide 'proper' and timely meals. Traces and suggestive implications of the same associations can be found in many published ethnographic accounts. In fact, conflict over meals as an occasion for domestic violence appears to be almost as ubiquitous as rituals of domestic food allocation.

Ellis points out that sociologists or policy makers often use the word 'trivial' to describe incidents of this kind which lead to brutality. She argues that insofar as 'in the men's eyes these apparently minor faults are seen as major crimes deserving punishment', they cannot be written off as unimportant. Ellis has got hold of a significant point here. Clearly these are not trivial issues. But the language of rights and contracts with which she goes on to discuss what is at issue seems inappropriate: 'One argument is that the men expect personal domestic service exclusive to them done only by their wives, and feel the marital contract is broken if this is not forthcoming.' The point is, of course, precisely that the basis on which exchanges take place in families is *not* a contract, but subject to a very different range of values and, indeed, feelings.

Although at one level the UK illustrations suggest that the demands for meals and food may symbolize the wider right to command and control which husbands are asserting, there are many more things at stake. Questions of femininity and masculinity, of love, of family life, of how needs are prioritized as well as the difficulties of male/female interdependence, are all raised by meals, by food and by cooking.

In this regard, it is important that power does not lie all in one direction, so I want to conclude with another example from the Ecuadorean community. Weismantel emphasizes that if the wife is supposed to serve food to her husband, reciprocally he is supposed to eat it and that this can become a weapon. She recalls how a young married couple travelled down the mountain to enjoy a fiesta, as they had done as a courting and newly married couple, but now they had a nursing infant and a toddler. As the day wore on, the wife got tired and dispirited, burdened with the children, and her husband slipped away 'for a few minutes' and disappeared.

> After a difficult trip home carrying both sleeping babies, up steep slopes in the dark, the wife was very angry indeed. When her husband arrived home many hours later, drunk and ready for bed, she informed him that he must be very hungry; as an obedient wife, she had prepared a nice dinner for him. Almost unconscious, he forced himself to sit upright long enough to eat two enormous bowls of soup under her reproachful eyes.[15]

The next day, he had to consume three more elaborate meals she had made, although he could not keep the food down. 'She appeared to enjoy cooking for him very much that day.'

The example speaks for itself, and it echoes the role of my grandmother in my childhood home, and other examples where women use meals, food and cooking to control family members. This female control, however, has always to be seen in the context of the overall power relations between the sexes, of which those involved in food and cooking are only a part. As Weismantel says: 'To cook is to speak and to mean, as well as to make and to do.' In cooking, it is women who are speaking, and what I have tried to show is that what is spoken and what is meant is complex, deep-rooted and often quite contradictory. It contains elements of servitude, of power, of affection, of imposed and willingly embraced altruism, of self-denial and of cheerful giving.

NOTES

1 *Saturday Night and Sunday Morning*, directed by Karel Reisz, 1961. Sex and moral issues, such as unmarried pregnancy and abortion, were treated more explicitly in this film than had been the case hitherto, and in ways which reflected many people's experience. But its success also came from the social realism with which it treated working-class life. Although this social realism looks very stereotyped from the vantage point of the 1990s, it was a breath of radical fresh air compared to the way class had been treated in British cinematic representation up until then.

2 *Manmade Famine*, Concord Films Council Ltd.
3 'The Mehanicu', Disappearing World Series, Granada, 1974.
4 Weismantel, M. (1988) *Food, Gender and Poverty in the Ecuadorian Andes*, Philadelphia, University of Pennsylvania Press.
5 Kerr, M. and Charles, N. (1988) *Women, Food and Families*, Manchester, Manchester University Press.
6 Harriss, B. (1991) 'The intrafamily distribution of hunger in South Asia', in J. Drèze and A. K. Sen (eds) *The Political Economy of Hunger* Vol. 1, London, Oxford University Press, pp. 351–424.
7 Harriss, 'Intrafamily distribution of hunger', p. 409.
8 Kerr and Charles, *Women, Food and Families*.
9 Murcott, A. (1985) 'On the social significance of the cooked dinner in South Wales', *Social Science Information* 21, 4–5; Murcott, A. (ed.) (1983) *The Sociology of Food and Eating*, Aldershot, Gower.
10 Both studies stress that their research was on both middle-class and working-class families.
11 Whitehead, A. (1981) 'I'm hungry mum', in K. Young et al. (eds) *Of Marriage and the Market*, London, Zed Press.
12 Whitehead, 'I'm hungry mum'.
13 Ellis, R. (1983) 'The way to a man's heart: food in the violent home', in Murcott (ed.) *The Sociology of Food and Eating*.
14 Kerr and Charles, *Women, Food and Families*.
15 Weismantel, *Food, Gender and Poverty in the Ecuadorian Andes*.

8

Food Production and Poverty

Michael Lipton

I

Are there strong links between poverty, inadequate food production and inadequate food consumption? Common sense suggests that, whenever a person (family, country) produces enough food staples, then – because rich people do not consume many more staples than poor people – that person (family, country) will tend to consume enough food; and that, whenever that happens, food poverty is banished. Of course, cities and city-states do not grow much of what they eat; nor do factory workers (or owners). But most poor countries, and poor people within them whether farmers or rural workers, do. For such people – even if a significant proportion of them works on non-farm activities,[1] or grows cash crops – 'food security' suggests that some steps need to be taken by them to avoid disaster in the event of failure of cash-crop harvests or prices, and to avoid complete reliance on long-distance purchases of food staples (with their usually high content of transport-and-trading costs). This usually means some involvement in food growing. The 'home gardens' of rubber smallholders and estate workers in Sri Lanka or Malaysia – and of rural, and even urban, non-farm workers in most developing countries – testify to this.

The production and consumption of enough food, and the absence of poverty, would thus appear to be rather closely linked. Yet the new conventional wisdom rejects this view for reasons explained later. It is generally believed that there is many a slip between producing enough food and having enough to eat, and between either of these and ending poverty: many a slip 'twixt cup and lip.

In fact this is one of many unlikely proverbs and quotations. There is seldom a slip 'twixt cup and lip.[2] I shall argue here that high rates of growth of staple food production, of staple food consumption relative to requirements, and of poverty reduction – while not necessary or sufficient for one another – are very strongly related, empirically and causally. For poor and/or rural areas, this normally applies at every level of aggregation. The individual, the household, the village, the region, the nation, that produces enough food (or raises the rate of food production sufficiently) will usually experience adequate, or improving, food consumption, and low, or falling, poverty.[3]

Let us start by defining the three concepts: being poor, not producing enough food, and not getting enough to eat. 'Being poor', in the absolute sense, means having too few resources to command the needs of life; in the extreme case too few resources to eat enough.[4] 'Not producing enough food' means producing too little food to eat enough – given one's other sources of claims upon food, and given one's ability to retain the income generated by one's non-food product (for example from net sales, or as wages) so as to convert it into food. So 'not producing enough food' means producing too little to avoid poverty, and in extreme cases to avoid getting 'too little to eat'. This is, however, a complex notion. 'Too little' means not enough to meet the needs (1) of an individual basal metabolic rate; (2) of work, including the work needed to produce and process, or to obtain, food; (3) for fighting off infections and parasites; and (4) of growth, reproduction, and for adult women of pregnancy and lactation. In all these cases, the levels of nutrient 'requirements' are controversial, context-dependent, and intercorrelated. Most are set according to body weight, and several vary with the individual's capacity to adjust to stress, or even with environmental temperature.

It is broadly true that, if people do not get enough to eat because they are poor, then it is because poverty is leading them to consume too few *calories* to meet their requirements. Of people who get sufficient calories, the great majority also get sufficient protein.[5] Micronutrient deficiencies – vitamin A and so on – are indeed important; however, such deficiencies are much less concentrated upon the poor (and much likelier to be cost-effectively treated by publicly mediated consumption, for example via the fortification of salt or sugar, rather than by extra privately purchased food intake), than is the case with calorie inadequacy. Therefore, if we are talking about not getting enough to eat in the sense that is linked to poverty, we are talking principally about not getting enough dietary energy – measured in joules, or, more familiarly, in (kilo) calories.[6]

How are poverty, inadequate food production and inadequate food consumption related? It is easiest to start by looking at this at an individual level: the level of Robinson Crusoe on his desert island, to revert to an old-fashioned style of doing economics. If Crusoe is very poor, he has too few resources to produce enough food – by hunting, gathering, fishing, agriculture and animal husbandry. Therefore he does not eat enough. Maybe the island is too small, the water scarce or ill-distributed, the terrain too rough, or the soil short of critical nutrients. In that simple case, presence of poverty, inability to produce enough food and incapacity to eat 'enough' amount almost to the same thing. Certainly the three are very closely related and causally interlinked; often each is necessary and sufficient for the others.

Yet some problems, familiar in real-life economies with many persons, also arise at the Crusoe level. Food availability year-round may be adequate but highly seasonal; can Crusoe store enough between seasons? Has he enough not only to eat, but also to put by for seed for next year? To sustain the working animals, if any? To handle likely levels of waste and storage losses? Crusoe also faces the problem of sustainability. Is he farming, hunting, and so on, in such a way that the adequacy of his food supplies will not diminish from one year to the next?

Despite such questions, it is clear that, at the Crusoe level, food production, food consumption and lack of poverty are very tightly linked. However, delinking becomes more likely even if we move a small step towards many-person real life: from a desert island with Crusoe to a desert island with a 'Swiss Family Robinson'. Adequate food production can be delinked from adequate food consumption, because the family as a whole may produce enough to eat, but may discriminate in allocation within the household, for example against women or children, so they do not obtain enough. Members of the Robinson household – unlike Crusoe – may have insufficient claims on food, even though food production (together with net 'imports') provides sufficient food availability for the family to eat enough in principle.

Conversely (and more benignly) a Robinson family member has a good chance of being cared for by his kin, whereas if Crusoe is old or ill he is likely to starve.

Also, families, as opposed to individuals, have new problems, and new prospects, affecting the nexus between poverty avoidance, 'enough' food to eat, and 'enough' food production. Unlike Crusoe, the family may contain children who need to grow, a mother who may need extra nutrients for pregnancy and lactation, and dependent elderly people. The family also has new prospects, unavailable to Crusoe, to produce – and to prepare for consumption – more food with less work and hence fewer energy requirements. Different family members can specialize, each in what she or he does best; and there may be scale economies, in production or in consumption, just because there is more than one person around.[7] Yet, even for the Robinson family, there is not much slippage between cup and lip. More food production, less poverty and more adequate food consumption are likely to move in lock-step most of the time. But what happens in a modern exchange economy?

There, it is pretty clear that producing enough food is neither necessary nor sufficient for consuming enough food. A person or family may produce no food at all, yet earn enough money (by producing other things) to obtain 'exchange entitlements', as Sen calls them, sufficient for all the food required.[8] Or a family may eat yet not work, thanks to inheritance or to 'social security'. On the other hand, a very poor family may produce lots of food, yet have to surrender so much that there is too little left for its own food needs: in an extreme case to a slave-owner, or, less extremely, to a landlord who takes a large share of a small crop. Or a small farmer may be forced to sell almost all his crop, at a low price after the harvest, to repay a debt – and may need to buy it back in the off season at much higher prices; such a family may produce lots of food, yet go hungry.

Such facts seem to delink food production, food consumption and poverty in modern exchange economies. A further empirical result deepens the questioning. Several recent studies[9] suggest that even quite poor people, when their incomes grow, do not make major increases in their calorie intake. They choose to spend their income on other things. So can these poor people be 'short of food' in a sense to which more food production would even be relevant?

Moving to the international level, we find another challenge to the commonsense linkages. Entire countries, in an exchange economy with international trade, appear able to delink food production from the attack on poverty and hunger. An economy like Hong Kong can almost end serious poverty, export its services and textiles to other countries, and enable almost all its citizens to consume enough food while the country produces hardly any food at all. Even 'successful' developing countries with big rural sectors, especially in East Asia but also in Latin America, have featured declining poverty and rising food consumption, hand-in-hand with declining food production and rising food imports. The poor have been eating better, switching away from food production, producing services and manufactured exports instead; their higher incomes have been used to import more food.

There is thus now a new conventional wisdom. Not only are poverty and hunger usually about inadequate entitlements to food (as Sen shows), but also food production, food consumption and poverty really have rather little to do with one another (as Sen has never alleged). I want to challenge this latter view.

First, with regard to the lack of linkage between poverty reduction and increased food consumption, wrong inferences have been drawn from studies showing that extra individual income has less impact than had been thought upon calorie intake. The main reason for this result, I believe, is that – when very poor people get a bit richer – their requirements of food often go down, because they reduce the large amount of overwork that they were doing. Although they may not greatly raise calorie intake when income rises, therefore, the relationship between the calories they get and the calories they spend in activity becomes more favourable. It is almost inconceivable that genuinely poor and hungry persons, when they get a bit better off, will not use a quite substantial part of their extra income in improving the balance between food intake and food requirements.

What about the alleged lack of linkage between levels of food production and adequacy of food consumption? Whether I go hungry or not is indeed determined by my entitlements to food – entitlements by exchange or in some other way – rather than by my or my nation's food production or even availability. But for most poor people in most poor places – not in Hong Kong, nor in Bombay – it is mainly food production itself that determines food entitlement. The large majority of the world's poor and hungry still depend on food production for income – either as employees on other people's food farms, or as producers of food on own-account. Since 1960 it has been to a considerable extent progress in the labour-intensive production of staple foodstuffs that pushed back hunger in many parts of Asia and Latin America; and absent or sluggish progress in food production that has caused the deepening crisis of poverty in sub-Saharan Africa.

We must also question the view, again rapidly becoming conventional, that fast growth in food output and productivity is delinked from poverty reduction (and from more adequate food consumption) because such growth is likely to succumb to the results of population growth, allegedly leading – alongside more intensive farming – to soil and water depletion or pollution: that the process is not sustainable. On the contrary, the main paths to growing more food – better availability and management of water, terrain, soil nutrients, and plant type and diversity – are also the essential paths to sustainability of natural resources. Moreover, widespread growth of incomes generally leads, not, as Malthus' early writings predicted, to more rapid population increase, but to improved prospects for child survival, for the education of children and adults, for parents' old-age security and for women's work. Such prospects frequently persuade parents to have fewer children.

High-input, high-output farming for the rapid growth of food output – and the higher food consumption (and demographic changes) induced – are keys to, not threats to, sustainable land and water use. On the other hand, so-called 'low-input, high-output agriculture' is a euphemism for mining away those soil and water resources. And 'low-input, low-output agricultures' are not going to make a sufficient dent either on poverty with populations growing at 2–3 per cent a year, or on the threats to sustainable agriculture as people respond in desperation and without substantially new and appropriate technology, to such population increase.

Despite this urgent need for new, high-input, high-output farming technologies – and despite their great successes in Asia – agricultural research into main food crops is being starved of essential public funding. During the 1980s, in sub-Saharan Africa and much of Latin America, national governments were faced by fiscal crises, and at the same time by pressures against state activity from aid donors. These governments have drastically reduced – and, especially in fiscal crises, destabilized – spending on food crop research. Even aid-funded international agricultural research spending, in the main institutes researching staple food crops, has gone down by over 10 per cent in real terms since the early 1990s, after stagnating for the previous decade.

As a result of these things, many people will die needlessly in the next 20 years. Hamlet urges Gertrude: 'Lay not that flattering unction to your soul / That not your trespass but my madness speaks'. In assessing Western parsimony in supporting staple food research,[10] we should not falsely comfort ourselves that – because Africans starve for want of food entitlements – we need not bother about the things that we in the West are doing to make Third World food production, and hence availability, grow needlessly slowly. More research to raise yields – and robustness, especially under moisture stress – of main tropical food staples could have prevented many deaths, especially in Africa, in the 1980s. Such food staples, especially if farmed labour-intensively, involve entitlements to food for the workers who grow them. High-yielding varieties in many parts of Asia have meant food that is more plentiful, cheaper and more reliably produced at the local level. These food staples are the means to saving lives and to reducing the poverty of those that remain alive to enjoy them.[11]

II

There are four main issues to be addressed here. I have already looked at the first: the *logic* of the relationships between being poor, not consuming enough food and not producing enough food; but more needs to be said about that later in the chapter. Second, it is necessary to review levels and trends of relevant food production, that is, production of food staples in developing countries, in the last thirty years or so, and ask what can be done for the less successful crops and areas. Third, we need to look at the levels and trends of absolute poverty, and at some of the characteristics of poor people. Fourth, in the light of the connections between trends in long-term food production and in absolute poverty – including the role of population growth and ecological decline in that linkage – we need to consider the role of policy.

First, what of the linkage between food production and absolute poverty? Let us start by looking at the poorer half of the populations of South Asia, East Asia and sub-Saharan Africa. These people are typically devoting at least 70–75 per cent of all their income to food. They have not sufficient income to save, or to spend on long-term objectives such as education, significantly. They can just about keep in the same place. Of these

Table 8.1 Food and sources, 1984–6

Country	*84–6 ppn (m)*	*Calories/ person/ day*	*% of calories from: roots tubers*	*cereals*	*Which main sources? (%)*
DCs		3400	4	30	
LDCs		2442	61	6	
Nigeria	95	2060	30	44	Sorghum 15, sweet potatoes 16, cassava 12, millet 12, maize 6, rice 6, wheat 4
Zaire	31	2124	57	16	Cassava 54
Sudan	22	2048	1	48	Sorghum 30, wheat 11
India	770	2143	2	63	Wheat 20, rice 30
China	1040	2622	7	71	Wheat 22, rice 38
Brazil	136	2667	7	39	Wheat 13, rice 15, maize 10

DCs: developed countries; LDCs: less developed countries

The data have many problems. (1) They are daily averages, over three years and all persons. They thus conceal problems due to unequal distribution of available calories over time, and among persons. (2) They are derived from data for food output, imports, exports and domestic seed, *feed*, *waste* and *changes in public and private stocks*; the data in italics are subject to large, shifting and uncertain margins of error – especially for small farmers in Africa, whose outputs are also estimated very unreliably (see footnote to table 8.3). (3) For DCs, the data refer to populations with much smaller proportions of infants and small children, and therefore considerably higher daily energy (calorie) requirements per average person, than in LDCs.

Source: FAO, *Food Balance Sheets*.

people, the large majority spend most of their working lives producing food staples, either as small farmers or, increasingly, as farm labourers.

Table 8.1 shows the average amount and composition of food intake. Because poor people have the lowest chances to diversify their diets, table 8.1 underestimates the extent to which food staples also dominate the consumption of poor people in the developing world. Typically, over 75 per cent of their calorie intake comes from five major cereals (wheat, rice, millet, maize and sorghum) and three root crops (yams, sweet potatoes and cassava). A typical member of the world's poor (1) spends most of his or her time – increasingly, as an employee rather than as a farmer – growing one or (less often) two of these eight food staples; and (2) derives most calorie intake from them. Ample, reliable, labour-intensively produced food staples are the key to the welfare of these people.

Even rural non-farm production is linked strongly to production of food staples. When such production increases, people in rural areas normally become wealthier, and better able to buy the crafts and services produced by other rural people. So the development of the whole rural economy is closely linked to what happens to food staples.

The 'poorer half' in India, China and Africa usually cannot save, but many of them have more or less enough to eat. However, the poorest 15 per cent or so of the populations of Asia and Africa are food-poor (ultra-poor). These people use at least 80 per cent of their income – including the self-consumed income which some of them produce on their own farms – to obtain food. Yet they eat at least 20 per cent less than the average daily requirements for age, sex and activity level laid down by the Food and Agriculture Organization (FAO) and the World Health Organization (WHO).[12] The data suggest that these ultra-poor people suffer sharply higher infant and child mortality, raised risks of being unable to perform as workers in adulthood, and possibly, although this is controversial, increased risk of mental inadequacies in surviving infants and children, than others. These dangers apply only to the ultra-poor, not to the moderately poor.[13]

Food staples production, then, is relevant to poverty most obviously because of (1) the high average proportion of income spent on food staples by the poor and the ultra-poor; (2) the high concentration of poor and ultra-poor people in food-growing places and jobs – so that extra discretionary income, made possible by food adequacy, is needed to enable such people to spend on other things than food, and to permit the economies to diversify and grow, as the domestic demand for new industries and crafts develops.[14]

Of course, the nutritional status (and discretionary income) of the poor may be most cost-effectively improved, not by pumping more food into them, but by improving their health levels or lowering their work requirements. Normally, however – to reduce poverty substantially where a lot of poor people are depending on food for both income and labour, and where particular food staples, which they themselves are producing, loom very large in their diets, but are eaten in insufficient quantities – food production per person in those regions has to increase.

III

Table 8.1 shows the disparity in the sources of food staples among people in various developing countries. Note that calories per person per day are much lower in the developing than in the developed world: 2,442 and

3,400 respectively (even though the need for dietary energy to fight off diseases and to provide fuel for physical work is substantially more in developing than developed countries). However, that disparity is less than it seems, because a much larger proportion of developing country populations consists of infants and small children who have lower calorie requirements, and because most Third World adults have less lean body mass to feed; these facts account for about two-thirds of the difference. But there remains a genuine shortfall in energy intake for many people in the developing world – reflected in infant and child mortality rates. Infant mortality rates are frequently as high as 150–200 per thousand. The balance of evidence is that about one in three of these infants dies partly because its body has been so weakened by undernutrition that it is unable to resist the onslaught of repeated infections.

Now consider the enormous difference in the calorie-mix in table 8.1. In the developed world we obtain only about one-third of our calories from staples: cereals, roots and tubers. In the developing world it is nearly two-thirds, and for the 'poorer half' of the people over three-quarters. Note also the huge differences within the developing world: sub-Saharan Africa is relatively dependent on roots and tubers; Asia and Latin America, on cereals. Within the cereals, for South and East Asia rice is still much the most important, but the huge rise in wheat yields in the 'green revolution' – and hence the relative cheapening of wheat – has increased its role in both production and consumption. In South and Central America, maize and wheat, and to some extent rice, are the main staples. Sub-Saharan Africa depends on roots and tubers for its calories almost as much as on cereals; the main cereals consumed, as well as grown, remain maize, millet and sorghum.[15] The typical African food staples are usually consumed near the place where they are produced; they have a low ratio of value to weight, that is, high transport costs per calorie, and they are well suited to most African lands.

That is important, in our consideration of the relationship between food production and hunger. Maize hybrids have displaced millet and sorghum in much of Africa – somewhat improving yields, but greatly increasing the vulnerability of production to drought. Even for maize, and especially for millets and sorghum, the rate of progress in yield enhancement has been much slower than for wheat and rice – particularly in sub-Saharan Africa, and in areas where water supply is insecure. In the root and tuber crops, progress has been slower still. The crops that had a 'green revolution' are rice and wheat, especially in adequately watered areas.

There are signs of progress in some of the other crops, notably hybrid sorghum and finger millet – progress mostly in India, but beginning to spread to other parts of the world, notably Zimbabwe. All the same, the great concentration of agricultural progress in 1964–80 that we call the green revolution – unquestionably the fastest change, over the widest area, ever to have happened to global food production – was very heavily concentrated on a small number of the crops, and growing conditions, in which the poor of the developing world operate. These crops and growing conditions are usually connected with the capacity to control one's water environment. This is physically impossible for most farmers in sub-Saharan Africa.[16]

We have seen that, for most people in most poor countries, the production of main food staples is closely linked to the adequacy of food consumption and to poverty reduction. However, such production has shown a disappointing performance for some of the main staples on which the poorest depend: roots and tubers; and coarse grains such as millets, sorghum and, to a lesser extent, maize.

Table 8.2 shows the performance of rice and wheat. These crops comprise only about 14 per cent of the area in sub-Saharan Africa that grows food staples, as opposed to two-thirds in the Far East and one-third in Latin America. For rice and wheat, shorter varieties of plant – which can be fertilized heavily without falling over – have been developed. In huge areas of tropical and sub-tropical wetlands, yields have been increased by a factor of two or even three since the mid-1960s.

In the early days of the 'green revolution', around 1965–73, it was widely feared that only the richer farmers would benefit. Since then, there has been substantial penetration of benefits, not only to very small farmers (though they adopted rather later), but also to landless labourers. Employment has been pulled up by the rise in staples crop production. Sometimes, this even helped the poor in regions 'left out' by the green revolution: landless labourers from such areas (such as parts of Bihar and Eastern Uttar Pradesh in India) not only enjoyed less expensive and more reliable food supplies, but were able to earn more 'entitlements' because they could migrate, for harvest work, to the green revolution areas such as the Indian Punjab. But, on the whole, poor people in areas where the green revolution has not happened have not done well. The higher yields in green revolution areas have restrained farm prices, and hence agricultural returns, for the rest of the developing world. Even table 8.2 hints at the big differences in yield for rice and wheat, among parts of the developing world. These differences depend substantially on water control, and hence on farmers' confidence to apply fertilizers and select the varieties that respond well to them. In 1987–8, the weight of plant nutrients from fertilizer, per average cropped hectare, was seven times more in India than in Africa, and in China it was 31 times more.

The impact of the best modern crop varieties can be seen by contrasting Sri Lanka and Sierra Leone, two countries where rice is the main food staple. In the early 1960s, rice in Sierra Leone and in Sri Lanka had much the same average yield, about one ton per hectare. Today, Sri Lanka's rice yield has tripled, mainly because reasonable security of water has encouraged farmers

Table 8.2 Rice and wheat

Region	*Area 1988–90 (m ha)*	*Yield 1988–90 (tons/ha)*	*Yield growth 1961–5/1988–90 (%)*
Rice			
Developed countries	4.4	5.8	18.4
Sub-Saharan Africa	5.3	1.6	26.6
Latin America	7.3	2.5	45.1
Far East	128.4	3.5	80.0
(China)	32.8	5.5	97.8
(India)	41.9	2.6	77.7
Wheat			
Developed countries	125.2	2.6	90.4
Sub-Saharan Africa	5.4	1.3	81.4
Latin America	10.7	2.0	41.3
Near East	21.2	1.6	65.7
Far East	62.6	2.5	188.5
(China)	29.6	3.1	247.3
(India)	23.5	2.1	155.4

Figures are three-year (or, for 1961–5, five-year) unweighted averages. 'Near East' is West Asia and North Africa.

Source: FAO, *Production Yearbooks* and *Quarterly Bulletins of Statistics*: latest available data for each year.

to adopt steadily improving rice varieties, initially tallish but robust cultivars bred from older stock, but, increasingly, carefully crossbred semi-dwarf plants, which can be much more heavily fertilized without falling over. Sierra Leone's average rice yield, however, is no higher now than thirty years ago.

Table 8.2 shows how these facts work out globally. Rice yields in sub-Saharan Africa average only 1.6 tons per hectare, as against 3.5 t/ha in the Far East – 5.5 t/ha in China. For wheat, the contrast is similar: though the few parts of Africa favourable for wheat – heavily concentrated in a few countries, notably the Sudan – have raised yields, these average only 1.3 t/ha in sub-Saharan Africa, as against 3.1 t/ha in China and 2.1 t/ha in India. But China and India have raised wheat yields dramatically only in the (substantial) areas that enjoy reasonable water security or control, and the fertilizers and semi-dwarf varieties that water management makes possible.

Even in parts of sub-Saharan Africa, rice and wheat varieties have improved substantially since the early 1970s. However, most of sub-Saharan Africa is stuck with crops where progress has been slower. Indeed, many areas lack the conditions of terrain, temperature or water to take full advantage of the possibilities of rice and wheat. Many cash crops – and, to some extent, even rapid progress with maize – also depend on much better water management.

This is not an argument for big dams all over sub-Saharan Africa. These have, on the whole and with a few striking exceptions (perhaps Gezira in the Sudan and Mwea in Kenya), proved uneconomic. They tend to cost three or four times as much, per hectare irrigated, as in South Asia (although the reason why is far from clear). Yet a population growing at typical African rates (2 per cent to $3\frac{1}{2}$ per cent a year, even more in some countries), and, except in a few special cases, running out of extra land, needs higher crop yields. These will grow much too slowly unless there is improved water control and water management. That will occasionally mean large-scale, bureaucrat-managed irrigation systems. However, in Asia as well as Africa, such schemes are running into increasing difficulties and decreasing returns. Normally, better water control in Africa requires small-scale, farmer-controlled irrigation systems, often modelled on the traditional techniques of the farmers themselves: valley-bottom irrigation, use of sand-rivers, small stream diversions.

Apart from raising the area irrigated from the present 3 per cent of cropland to, say, 10 per cent in the next 10–15 years, sub-Saharan Africa requires a major push to increase yields of crops on rainfed land, and their robustness under moisture stress, by varietal research in its main food staples. Otherwise, most of Africa, which comprises the semi-arid regions in which such crops grow, will continue the trends of 1960–90: a substantial decline in food availability per person, which (in view of the rapid rise in food imports) implies an even faster decline in food production per person. Table 8.3 shows both that sub-Saharan Africa is much more dependent on the largely rainfed staples than the other continents, and – very importantly – that even in these crops, Africa's yield improvement has been relatively slow.[17]

Food production in sub-Saharan Africa is not constrained *only* by lack of water control, even together with inadequate research into its main crops. Many people have correctly drawn attention to price policies biased against food crops and against farmers who grow them. However, the response to price improvements for the agricultural sector as a whole in sub-Saharan Africa has been weak and disappointing. For an individual crop, if the price rises farmers will grow more of it by shifting productive resources from other crops. But if the prices of all farm crops rise – relative to, say, land prices, or the price of consumer goods like clothes or houses – there is not a lot that farmers can do, unless improved technologies are available. They

Table 8.3 Millet, sorghum, maize, roots and tubers

Region	*Area 1988–90 (m ha)*	*Yield 1988–90 (tons/ha)*	*Yield growth 1961–5/1988–90 (%)*
Millet			
Developed countries	3.0	1.31	+ 81.9
Sub-Saharan Africa	13.1	0.66	+ 31.0
Far East	20.2	0.79	+ 41.0?
(India)	16.6	0.67	+ 63.0
Sorghum			
Developed countries	5.1	3.40	+ 27.3
Sub-Saharan Africa	13.8	0.81	+ 15.7
Near East	5.0	0.72	– 14.0
Far East	17.4	1.01	+106.0
(India)	14.9	0.70	+ 79.0
Maize			
Developed countries	45.5	5.6	+ 77.0
Sub-Saharan Africa	16.8	1.2	+ 37.0
Latin America	26.3	2.0	+ 59.0
Far East	38.1	3.0	+ 78.0
(China)	20.4	4.0	+ 61.0
(India)	5.9	1.5	+ 56.0
Roots, tubers			
Developed countries	11.8	16.6	+ 25.8
Sub-Saharan Africa	14.7	7.6	+ 24.6
Latin America	4.2	11.4	+ 8.6
Far East	18.7	11.9	+ 45.1
(China)	12.2	11.7	+ 38.0
(India)	1.3	15.6	+ 43.0

All data for roots and tubers are affected by the difficulty of estimating output for crops often left long in the ground and harvested according to need, if at all. African data – especially for roots and tubers; in many countries also for millet and sorghum, less so for maize – are highly unreliable, due to data-gathering deficiencies, and to the variable or unclear treatment of mixed cropping. Chinese data for millet (and perhaps sorghum) yield growth are highly unreliable, because a large area of low-yielding millet (and a significant area of sorghum) 'disappeared' from the statistics in 1968–72, probably due to reclassification.

Source: FAO, *Production Yearbooks* and *Quarterly Bulletins of Statistics*: latest available data for each year.

generally have not been available for coarse grains and tubers on unreliably watered, semi-arid or humid lands in sub-Saharan Africa.

This ultimate constraint in Africa – on raising production of food staples and on raising poor farmers' and farmworkers' income-based entitlements to their consumption, and therefore on reducing extreme poverty – cannot be lifted only by 'policy dialogue', or by aid conditioned upon getting price or foreign-exchange policies right. Unless something is done about the acquisition (as well as the generation) of agricultural technology, not much will happen. Many institutions seek to do something about this. The Consultative Group for International Agricultural Research now spends almost half its $300-odd million yearly outlays on, and usually in, sub-Saharan Africa. But the impact of such efforts depends on applied research in what are termed '*National* Agricultural Research Systems'. Unfortunately, most of these in Africa have been weakly and unreliably funded by national governments. Total – domestic plus aid-financed – agricultural research spending per farmer, or per hectare, or per dollar's worth of agricultural output, in a typical year is actually higher in sub-Saharan Africa than in either of the other two developing continents.[18] But that money currently has low productivity. African agricultural research is exceptionally badly related to cropping patterns, and tends especially to neglect roots, tubers, millet and sorghum. Also, in Africa it costs more to pay each scientist than in other developing countries – yet each scientist produces less 'output'.[19] The main reason for this low research productivity is the rapid turnover of national (and expatriate) scientists, in circumstances where research prospects are limited by the extreme unreliability of funding for the nationally funded parts of agricultural research.

The numbers for food output in Africa are also pretty unreliable – a sign, alongside the willingness of politicians to slash national agricultural research budgets when cash becomes scarce, of the low prestige of agriculture, and the low expectations and political impact of rural people. However, it is indisputable that food staples production per person in most of Africa has fallen sharply since 1960. Imports have risen at faster rates than population growth, yet the incidence of undernutrition has not declined. Not only have research results – and yield gains – in the main food crops on which three out of four of the African poor depend for livelihoods been globally worse than for rice and wheat; such results have been specially bad in Africa, because of unreliable water and unreliable research support.

In this situation, it has been argued that farmers in poor areas should migrate, leave agriculture, or at least stop growing 'traditional' crops and just grow wheat and rice. The latter has been tried, usually with disastrous results. The reason that cassava and sorghum are grown in many areas is that these crops are well adapted to rainfall pattern, soil structure and chemistry, pest population and terrain. If you try to force the wrong crops onto these areas you get bad results at very great cost.

What about moving out of agriculture altogether? Should Chad specialize, not in agriculture nor even in animal husbandry, but rather in some form of manufacturing output? Common sense casts doubt on such applications of the 'principle of least comparative disadvantage'. Where it has been tried, the main result has been to damage further what agricultural progress was taking place. There is overwhelming evidence that rural success in non-farm activities starts with growth in agriculture – and in consequent increases in local demand for tools, processing, and for consumer goods and services. Non-farm development does not readily happen where, let alone because, farming stagnates.

A third, radical, option has been migration. Of course some migration does happen out of the areas of stagnant crop yields, towards more progressive parts of sub-Saharan Africa: to places where hybrid maize is moving forward, in parts of Kenya, Malawi and Zimbabwe; to areas of success with cocoa and coffee, in parts of the Ivory Coast and Togo. Such migration, though, is a slow process; and generally there are special constraints on migration by the very poor.[20] Meanwhile, population growth in the stagnant areas continues.

Many of the developments in the advanced and well-watered areas of Asia and Africa have not made it easier to solve the problems of the 'backward' areas. Consider the potential solution of labour emigration. Recent agricultural growth has tended to employ less extra labour than before. In Asia, green revolution types of increase in rice or wheat yields on a farm that thereby produced 20 per cent more output in the mid-1970s brought some 8 per cent extra employment. Now, a similar yield increase brings only 3–4 per cent extra employment.[21] And the agrarian structure has also sometimes changed in ways harmful to employment (and therefore to immigration). Much of Africa, and some of Asia, has seen a concentration of ownership, either of land or of tractors or animals, especially within the better farming regions; and big farms use less labour, and more equipment and land, than do small farms in order to produce a given amount of output. So, paradoxically, after initially pulling in migrants from distant and backward areas, some of the best crop-growing areas, like the Comilla area in Bangladesh, have recently been expelling labour to fragile areas. It has become more difficult for migrants out of 'backward' rural areas to get work in more favourable farmlands, because of weedicides, tractors, reaper-binders, even in some cases combine harvesters, which have caused the net displacement of labour.

There are therefore areas such as the western desert of Rajasthan in India, and many areas in East Africa, where there is substantial net growth of population in spite of a very fragile and inadequate land and resource base; and the solution of voluntary large-scale migration from these areas (while to be encouraged if feasible) is not in practice likely to do much to help. These environmentally fragile arid and semi-arid areas of the developing world – not only in sub-Saharan Africa, but also in South Asia, China and to some extent Latin America – are now the heartlands of world poverty. They contain 35–45 per cent of the rural Third World's poor population (but only 20–5 per cent of its non-poor population).[22] It is self-deception to believe that the problems of these people can be solved *mainly* by a massive shift into new crops, by movement to non-agriculture, or by migration. The problems will largely remain: how to grow food in place, in a sustainable way by increasing productivity especially per hectare (but also per person) for the existing, largely neglected, rather unsatisfactory food crops[23] and how to provide more reliable water management or water control, so that small farmers can both produce more and employ landless workers in the process.

IV

I pass now from the question of food production, to the question of absolute poverty: the inability to afford a given minimum-needs basket, usually in practice measured in terms of food consumption per person. Relative poverty gives rise to misery and envy and is therefore bad, but it is a confusing concept because it mixes up poverty and inequality. I prefer to look at absolute poverty and inequality as separate issues, although both of them are important.

The severity of absolute poverty depends on three factors: the level of gross national product (GNP) per person; the distribution of GNP between higher- and lower-income receivers; and the distribution of income among persons with low income. The second item, share of GNP going to poor people, is closely related to relative poverty – which is, therefore, one component of absolute poverty. Nevertheless, it is principally absolute poverty that harms people, and at its extremes kills people.

Most attempts to measure absolute poverty are confined to private income or consumption. This makes us rather too pessimistic when we look at changes in poverty. In India, during a period when official measures of poverty improved very little, Jodha[24] showed that most people classified as poor felt that they had become much better off. This is mainly, I believe, because crude poverty data measure only private income and consumption, and lead to the question: is *that* enough to acquire a bundle of basic needs? The answer to that question misses – as the poor certainly do not – possible improvements in public-sector or community provision of basic health, primary education, even roads.

One further issue is that of chronic versus transient poverty. We now have several surveys which, for several years, have collected information about income or consumption each year from the same 'panel' of households. These 'panel data' suggest that about one in three of all households, found to be in income poverty at a given moment of survey, are 'transient': that is, at least half the time they are not poor. They drift in and out of poverty. The other two-thirds appear to be in more or less permanent poverty.

Transient poverty can be just as harmful as, or worse than, permanent poverty. A major cause of transient poverty is the presence of many small children, with only one adult available to earn money. For underfed infants, such transient poverty can be a killer. But it is a different sort of problem from that of permanent poverty and requires a different sort of treatment, whether through more stable employment income and food prices, or through social safety nets.

Unfortunately, most surveys do not measure who is transiently poor and who is permanently poor. They measure those who are in poverty at the time of the survey, in terms of private income or consumption. Yet such numbers (see table 8.4) are of considerable interest.

These numbers show how many people are below each of two poverty lines, a lower and a higher. Even the lower poverty line, $275 of constant purchasing power parity (PPP) per year in 1989, is still considerably above the level at which undernutrition normally appears – but note the 'gap': the average 'very poor' person is almost 10 per cent below this lower poverty

Table 8.4 World poverty, 1989: less developed countries (LDCs)

Region	*Population (millions)*	*$275 PPP per year: % below*	*% gap*	*$370 PPP per year: % below*	*% gap*
Sub-Saharan Africa	440	34.9	9.5	52.0	17.2
East Asia	1450	4.9	1.0	11.3	2.7
(China)	(1100)	(5.3)	(1.2)	(10.9)	(2.9)
South Asia	1130	27.6	6.2	49.3	14.6
(India)	(830)	(30.5)	(6.8)	(53.6)	(16.1)
Eastern Europe	70	3.4	0.8	6.9	1.9
Near East	210	21.1	5.5	33.1	9.6
Latin America, Caribbean	420	16.8	5.7	24.8	9.3
All LDCs	3740	17.5	4.3	30.3	9.1

PPP: purchasing power parity; 1985 dollars, Indian prices and consumption bundles. % gap is between income of the average per person and the stated poverty line, both in PPP dollars.

Source: Re-estimated by Martin Ravallion, from 1985 data in *World Development Report 1990* and more recent information. Data for 'all LDCs' include small items for areas not listed above.

line in Africa, and almost 7 per cent in India. Almost all the 'very poor' are severely stressed and miserable as a result of not having enough income, but some of them, perhaps 25–35 per cent, are not at risk of serious energy stress, and do not suffer infant and child mortality much, if at all, above the level which applies to the non-poor. For most of the group below the lower poverty line, however, health risks are significantly increased.

Table 8.4 gives two distinct poverty indicators (both for extreme and for moderate poverty): the percentage of persons below a poverty line, or the *incidence* of poverty; and the percentage gap between the average poor person and the poverty line, or the *intensity* of poverty (poverty gap). Such figures are important – not because of any journalistic or academic interest in counting the poor, or in scrabbling around and trying to find out about how poor they are, but rather for their significance in the effort to reduce poverty. To do that, one needs to know the dimensions of the problem. In a particular area, are there 10 per cent of the population who are 1 per cent below a given poverty line, or 1 per cent who are 10 per cent below it? Quite different public policy responses are appropriate. It does not suffice to know the incidence alone, that is, the percentage of people below the poverty line. We also need, at very least, some idea of the intensity – the poverty gap.

In table 8.4, note the low incidence and severity of poverty in Eastern Europe, especially of severe poverty. Only 3.4 per cent of the population are below the lower poverty line, and they average only 0.8 per cent below that line. We need to be wary about attempts to redirect international attention and aid away from the developing countries, towards areas where poverty is much less.

The proportions of the population who are subject to nutrition risk – that is, to a significantly higher probability of functional impairment due to inadequate nutrient (usually calorie) intake – as a result of low income in sub-Saharan Africa and South Asia is in the order of 17–22 per cent, as against 30–5 per cent beneath even the lower poverty line in table 8.4. The incidence of poverty is now somewhat higher in sub-Saharan Africa than in South Asia – a reversal of the situation of the early 1970s. Sub-Saharan African numbers are much less reliable than the others.[25] However, there is a lot of supporting evidence that the time trend of poverty has been much worse since 1970 in sub-Saharan Africa than elsewhere.

There have been some important changes in measured poverty. In India, a very large developing country, the incidence of poverty has fallen by a quarter between 1979 and 1989. Much more dramatic falls were seen elsewhere, notably in China. In Indonesia the incidence fell by two-thirds between 1970 and 1987. In Pakistan and in Thailand it fell by half. However, in sub-Saharan Africa the proportion in poverty is slightly higher now than it was in the 1960s, and has certainly risen since 1980; and in Latin America there has been, at best, no improvement since 1980.

We have some idea, through poverty profiles and village-level research, of who the poor are. Disaggregations of the above numbers, plus the poverty profiles, suggest further relationships between poverty, food consumption and food production. The poor are heavily concentrated in large families. Typically, 70 per cent of people below various national poverty lines are in families of six or more persons (as against about half of the non-poor). This is due mainly to very high ratios, in big families, of non-earning children to earning adults. Hence, of course, children are very heavily concentrated in the poor groups. Since it is in childhood that the damage done by inadequate food consumption is particularly great and sometimes irreversible, that creates a serious and special problem of child poverty.[26]

Although poverty is concentrated in large households, it is not specially concentrated in female-headed households or among women. Nevertheless, women are grossly disadvantaged in the developing world (as in some parts of the developed world). But the disadvantage does not consist in a greater risk of absolute poverty, but rather in the need for women – in order to obtain a level of living similar to men's – to work longer and harder, and with less hope of advancement. Women are expected not only to look after the house and the children and the cooking, but also to work in the fields. So they work longer hours. Also, they usually have much less access to education, and therefore to jobs at high incomes, than men.

However, when income gets pooled in the household, there is no evidence that women are more heavily concentrated in households in the poverty groups than are men. Yet there *is* maldistribution of calories within the households of a particular region of the world, against particular subsets of females: small girls aged between six months and three years. Therefore infant mortality (0–1 year), and, much more clearly, mortality between one and five years of age, is higher in girls, relative to boys, in this region than it need or should be.

The evidence for this is very localized. Barbara Harriss has shown that in South Asia the phenomenon of discrimination in energy distribution by gender is confined to parts of Pakistan, Bangladesh and Northern India. Peter Svedberg has shown that in sub-Saharan Africa the distribution of calorie intake, if anything, favours females.[27]

That is not surprising when gender divisions of work in production are unpacked. In Africa, women do most of the work in producing food. So, on a fairly crude model of food as investment, these desperate families (in trying to survive) are going to steer more calories, relative to requirements, towards the girls, who are tomorrow's producers. Contrariwise, in Northern India and Bangladesh – whether because of culture and custom, or because of the types of farmwork available – women are less involved in agricultural production pre-harvest and there is less agricultural demand for female farm labour. There, many households tend to steer more calories, relative to requirements, towards the male children. These are the terrible dilemmas produced by extreme poverty and lack of food adequacy, rather than (I think) consequences of male patriarchy at the level of the household.

This is a controversial issue. Certainly, there is discrimination against women in poor countries. But we need to be clear about the types and the reasons for it. Women are not, as a rule, poorer than men; but they have to work more, especially in the home, and with less hope of advancement, to achieve similar income levels.

That rural poverty exceeds urban poverty is less controversial. The numbers (for example in the World Bank's 1990 *World Development Report*) show this; but they do not show it, as it were, nearly enough. This is another effect of the fact that these data define poverty lines in terms of private income associated with a given level of satisfaction of needs (in particular, dietary energy requirements). Above, I pointed out that this gives too bleak a picture of change, because the big gain made by the poor in the Third World, in many countries, has been via access to public provision of health, education, roads and other needs. However, this public provision has been extremely unequal: heavily concentrated in urban areas, and especially sparse in remote areas. The rural–urban gaps in such indicators as infant mortality are really quite horrendous, and indicate a distribution of poverty much more unfavourable to the rural areas than the disparities in private income (or consumption) per person might suggest.

Consider the Ivory Coast, a West African country with unusually good surveys of household poverty. In the Ivory Coast, the proportion of people living in households below a 'poverty line' – of private income per person associated in a typical household with just-adequate calorie intake – in rural areas is 57 per cent, and in urban areas it is 46 per cent: not a very big difference. Yet rural infant mortality is 121 per 1000; urban infant mortality is 70 per 1000, an enormous difference.

In India, table 8.4 probably understates the difference between the proportions of rural and urban populations below a poverty line defined in terms of private income or consumption level alone;[28] but the urban advantage in private incomes is not huge. The lower average rural incomes are almost balanced in their effect on poverty incidence by the less unequal rural distribution. Yet, in 1985, 105 per 1000 of all rural children in India died before reaching the age of one, as against 57 per 1000 urban children. The latter is still a terribly high number, but is much lower than in rural areas, where birth hygiene, health facilities and the mother's chance of being attended by a trained midwife, in particular, are so much less than in the town.

In 1982, the Indian journal *Economic and Political Weekly* published a celebrated article called 'Little girls and death in India'.[29] This article showed that, compared with almost all other parts of the world, girls in Northern India had worse survival chances relative to boys. Almost certainly large numbers of Northern Indian girls are dying every year as a result of male–female discrimination – in food consumption and/or in health-care provision. This is indeed an avoidable tragedy. Yet, if there were an article called 'Young villagers and death', there would be about 15 times as many infant deaths to record as a result of the urban–rural disparity in infant mortality as are attributable to the gap between boys and girls. This urban–rural health disparity is primarily in 'public expenditure' against poverty – clean water, preventive health care at birth, inoculation, control of infection. These are missing in the villages to a much greater extent than in the urban areas – and this in a country, India, where there is great democratic pressure from below, where villagers are not speechless or powerless, and where a substantial attempt is made, within some centres of urban power, to correct these deficiencies.[30] Regional disparity is also great: within India, infant mortality in the southern rural areas was 78 per 1000 around 1985, as against 142 in central rural areas.[31]

V

What, then, is needed from policy makers in poor and rich countries to raise Third World food production in ways that reduce poverty? Recall that, though people have dealt with population growth for many millenia by expanding the area under food crops, the capacity for such a response was more or less exhausted by 1965 in South and East Asia, and by 1990 in much of Africa. Yield expansion therefore is going to be required to feed these extra people.

The key issue is: will the extra yield be generated in ways that allow the hungry to earn income and thus afford food? This is the true nature of the 'race' between population and food output: the extra food output has to run three-legged, alongside extra access (by potentially undernourished people) to income. The jobs, to earn the income to obtain the food, are likely, for reasons already given, to come mainly from agricultural production, especially food production itself.

However, although, if cropped area expands 10 per cent and output expands 10 per cent, jobs usually expand 10 per cent as well, the three-legged race is harder to run if output expansion depends not on extra area but on higher crop yields. If extra output is being obtained through yield expansion of 10 per cent, typically in the mid-1960s that raised labour use and employment by only 4 per cent. In the 1990s, for rice and wheat, the corresponding growth in labour input is even less – only about $1\frac{1}{2}$–2 per cent. That is because, alongside the high-yielding varieties, there have arrived inputs designed mainly for the requirements of the labour-saving, large-scale European and North American farmers, who provide the great bulk of the demand for agricultural research: tractors, weedicides, and so forth.

There is nothing wicked going on here. The ordinary operations of the market mean that research will be geared mainly to saving resources that are scarce for those who can afford research; but technology spreads beyond the borders for which it was initially intended. If tens of millions of dollars are spent to cut the cost of farming with tractors (thus saving, that is, unemploying, labour), but only tens of thousands of dollars on improving the efficiency of hoeing or animal-ploughing, then tractor-ploughing becomes more attractive, not only in the US and Europe, but also in India and Africa. Similarly with weedicides, relative to hand weeding. All this has the effect of not providing, on a world scale, enough demand for labour to enable the poor in Asia and Africa to obtain farm employment sufficient to afford the extra food that they need, even if that extra food is being grown.

Some economists talk of 'market failures' in these circumstances. These are not market failures; these are the unhappy and sometimes terrible consequences of market success.[32]

What can be done to make 'market success' more often a sentence of life, rather than death, for many of the world's poor? Agricultural research on national and international levels has in the past related, with frequently good poverty-reducing results, to farmers' requirements in water-controlled areas growing rice and wheat. Yield expansion has much more than replaced area expansion, as a source of output growth, since the mid-1960s in those areas. There is hardly any more arable area in the Indian Punjab to expand into, but wheat and rice yields have been growing faster than areas ever did, and yields have tripled since the mid-1960s. Really rapid growth of food production did create employment, both on the farms, and to meet the farmers' increasing demand for processing transport, housing, and so on.

Indeed, there is probably nowhere in the world where food output per inhabitant is growing at 2 per cent a year or more and poverty is not decreasing. Such a rapid growth of food output sets up extra demands for farm workers – and extra spending by farmers and farm workers creates further new demand for labour and helps push poverty down. Conversely, there is probably no significant rural area of the low-income developing world where food output per person is stagnating or declining, yet poverty is not increasing.

The poor are now heavily and increasingly concentrated in regions with no water control – regions that grow and eat mainly roots and tubers (in Africa) or coarse grains (in India). In India in 1972–3, the National Sample Survey divided the rural areas of India into 57 regions, and measured poverty (and many other things) there. In each of the ten regions with the lowest poverty incidence, fewer than 27 per cent of rural people were poor, and the proportion of cropland irrigated was 28 per cent. In the ten regions with most poverty, more than 60 per cent of people were poor, and only 6 per cent of all cropland areas was irrigated.[33]

Food adequacy is about entitlements, not 'output' as such; if food available to a country were distributed according to need, many fewer people would be hungry. But food entitlements are largely about being able to earn income from work. While some places can specialize in cash crops, animal production or non-farm activity, for the great bulk of the world's poor the amount of available work depends on the prosperity of food-growing agriculture, and in particular on increasing yields where land is becoming more scarce.

VI

It is not, in general, true that these processes in the long run will cause environmental degradation. Directly, careful water and nutrient management, including in many cases higher inputs of fertilizer and irrigation, stabilize and improve agricultural sustainability. Indirectly, more employment – to earn widely spread entitlements to an increasing output-per-person of food staples – has in many cases led to slower, not faster, population growth.

In Malthus' late work, notably the 1824 paper published as the entry on 'Population' in the 1830 edition of the *Encyclopaedia Britannica*, he noted the 'extreme healthiness' of several Swiss cantons, and used census data to show that, following declines in the death rate, couples had voluntarily taken action to reduce the birth rate, so that population was no longer growing rapidly. We are beginning to rediscover that widely shared modern economic growth, based on rising total factor productivity especially in labour-intensive food production, does not destroy environments by causing populations to explode, but creates possibilities for parents to have fewer children, yet to be reasonably sure of producing a surviving, healthy, perhaps educated successor, who will obtain work and support them in their old age.

Malthus also advocated universal education. Recent evidence has clearly shown that women's secondary and further education, in particular, brings down their desired family size (1) by delaying marriage; (2) by increasing the opportunity-cost of child-rearing (because educated women have better earnings prospects outside the home); (3) by improving mothers' skills in child care, so that fewer infants and small children die and are replaced by extra births; (4) by encouraging parents to have fewer but better-educated children (including girls) and thereby to 'substitute quality for quantity', and *perhaps* (5) by raising women's information about contraception, and the decision-taking power of women in the family *vis-à-vis* their husbands.

So demographic and environmental concerns, except in the very short term, are not a valid reason for the reduced shares of national and international expenditures on Third World agricultural research and investment,[34] and, in particular, for tolerating a deceleration of growth in Third World food output. We know what needs to be done by agricultural research. Of course, many of the under-researched crops and regions pose difficult problems for research. Researchers tend to do first the things that they know best how to do, and that safely offer a high return to research. That is natural and only right. But Bernard Shaw was not quite right when he wrote in *The Doctor's Dilemma*: 'Every profession is a conspiracy against the laity'. What every profession is a conspiracy against is, in fact, acceptance of the law of diminishing returns. We professionals like to do what we think or know we can do well. That is rewarded, not only with a sense of achievement and security, but also with publications, promotion, kudos. It is risky to research the areas where many have failed before. It is risky to work on root and tuber crops. So far, therefore, both efforts and results have been much greater for the top crops in the best-irrigated areas. What is needed is to get incentives and resources for national as well as international agricultural research systems to devote themselves far more to sustainable farming systems for the production of higher-yielding, and more moisture-stress-resistant, varieties of poor people's crops in the more difficult areas. The experience since the 1960s shows that it can be done. Finger millets and hybrid sorghums in India, and now in some parts of Africa, point the way. Far more such research needs to be done.

NOTES

1 Typically, a quarter of working time (and a third of income) in a developing rural area is non-farm.

2 G. M. Hopkins chided Wordsworth: 'The Child is father of the Man? / The Poet's words were wild! / The Man is father of the Child'. P. G. Wodehouse advised Duke Senior, in Shakespeare's *As You Like It*, to look for '*Stones* in the running brooks, / Sermons in *books*', rather than vice versa. Paul Streeten reminds us that probably nobody has ever killed two birds with one stone.

3 These statements are empirical and therefore falsifiable. One could, of course, readily define 'poverty, consumption, production' so as to make the statements into tautologies, but I shall not do so.

4 Strictly, some definition such as that of the Indian National Sample Survey is needed: an Indian household is below the 'poverty line' if it spends, per month, less than *would be* required to obtain enough dietary energy (calories) to feed its members 'enough' (see below), *if* it distributed its spending between food and other items, and among foods, in the 'average' way for households of its size, demographic structure, and total expenditure.

5 Most cereal staples contain 7 to 11 per cent protein, and in poor countries are both grown and eaten (note the linkage!) alongside protein-rich legumes; even with almost no animal foods, such consumption normally leads to a sufficiently balanced (and adequate) amino-acid intake, provided enough calories are ingested. Diets with root-crop staples can create protein problems, but (for example) cassava leaves – usually consumed as well as the roots – are quite rich in protein.

6 One (kilo) calorie is almost exactly 4.3 joules.

7 Farming, unless quite heavy mechanization is involved, seldom features economies of scale. However, cooking for two (or three) uses much less than two (or three) times as much fuel, or working time, as cooking for one.

8 Sen, A. K. (1981) *Poverty and Famines*, Oxford, Clarendon Press.

9 Behrman, J. 'Nutrition and incomes: tightly wedded or loosely meshed?', Pew Memorial Lecture, Cornell Food Policy Program, Ithaca, NY, 1988.

10 The same warning, against deceiving ourselves that we do not harm others because they are themselves to blame, applies to other Western behaviour that has damaged Third World food positions: agricultural policies, especially in Europe, that depress world prices and discourage Third World cereal production; monetary policies that raise world real interest rates and deter agricultural, especially resource-conserving, investment; and research incentives that produce labour-displacing bias in world technical progress.

11 See Mellor, J. and Desai, G. (eds) (1986) *Agricultural Change and Rural Poverty*, New Delhi, Oxford University Press, for clear evidence that the incidence of 'food poverty' in India is lower in places and times of (1) high agricultural output; (2) low prices of food staples.

12 Adult body weight (and probably basal metabolic rate) among poor sub-groups in LDCs is substantially below the 'Western' reference or average level; and ambient temperature is considerably higher. The upshot is that a shortfall of 10 per cent or even 15 per cent below Western 'average daily requirements' of calories (dietary energy) is probably not usually a danger signal for such subgroups.

13 Lipton, M. (1983) *Poverty, Undernutrition and Hunger*, Washington, DC, World Bank.

14 Such domestic demands, and the skills to meet them, are normally the basis for industries that later produce successful exports. This is not, however, an iron law – and is hardly ever a good reason for exchange-rate or protectionist policies that discriminate in favour of production for the home market, and therefore against exports.

15 Even in South and East Asia, though wheat and rice are the dominant urban foods, there are very large rural areas, particularly in China, where (very importantly) maize, to some extent sorghum, or even root crops, are the staple food. That is much more the case, however, in sub-Saharan Africa. The urban tendency to wheat and rice consumption impinges very heavily on politicians in Africa, but is much less widespread than one would guess to hear the policy discussions. It does not at all justify 'import-saving' via recent, very expensive rice-growing irrigation schemes in West Africa, or current attempts to grow wheat in totally unsuitable tropical areas in Central and Eastern Africa.

16 Barely 3 per cent of cropped area in sub-Saharan Africa is irrigated; in Asia it is about one-third.

17 Some economists argue that this is partly because African agricultures are usually short of labour (not land), and therefore have little incentive to adopt – or develop – yield-increasing methods. But since the early 1970s more and more African regions have run short of good, spare arable land. Also, the best way to save labour, per unit of output, is often by adopting improved varieties that save land. And, in any case, most of Africa has experienced declining food output per farm worker – not just per hectare – since the 1960s, relative to other developing areas and in some cases absolutely: Timmer, P. (1988) 'The agricultural transformation', in H. Chenery and T. N. Srinivasan (eds) *Handbook of Development Economics*, Vol. 1, Amsterdam, North-Holland.

18 Lipton, M. (1988) 'The place of agricultural research in the development of sub-Saharan Africa', *World Development* 16, 10.

19 How do you measure the output of a scientist? A weighted index of publications is used – not a wonderful measure, but the best available.

20 For evidence, see Connell, J., Dasgupta, B., Laishley, R. O. and Lipton, M. (1976) *Migration from Rural Areas: the evidence from Village Studies*, New Delhi, Oxford University Press.

21 Lipton, M. with Longhurst, R. (1989) *New Seeds and Poor People*, London, Unwin Hyman, ch. 4.

22 Estimates (for 1989) by the International Food Policy Research Institute, Washington, DC.

23 Cash crops (if tolerant of moisture stress) may provide substantial help. In practice, this usually depends on better communications and infrastructure than the 'traditionally backward' regions growing coarse grains, roots and tubers enjoy.

24 Jodha, N. S. (1989) 'Social science research on rural change: some gaps', in P. Bardhan (ed.) *Conversations between Economists and Anthropologists*, New Delhi, Oxford University Press.

25 For Latin America and South and East Asia, about 90 per cent of the populations who are reported on in table 8.4 are measured from household surveys. In sub-Saharan Africa it is only about 11 per cent. So the confidence intervals around these numbers are extremely wide. To give some notion, Martin Ravallion (who built this table) comments that, though 52 per cent of the population of sub-Saharan Africa, on the best estimate, are in 'moderate poverty', our 95 per cent confidence intervals are far apart, around that 52 per cent figure: namely, 17 per cent and 76 per cent (personal communication)! In other words, we are 95 per cent sure only that the proportion of sub-Saharan Africans in moderate poverty lies between 17 per cent and 76 per cent! We are much more confident about the numbers for the rest of the developing world.

26 Evidence for this and subsequent paragraphs is summarized in Lipton, M. (1988) *The Poor and the Poorest*, Washington, DC, World Bank.

27 Svedberg, P. (1990) 'Undernutrition in sub-Saharan Africa: is there a gender bias?', *Journal of Development Studies* 26, 3.

28 Minhas, B. S., Jain, L. R. and Tendulkar, S. D. (1991) 'Declining incidence of poverty in the 1980's: evidence versus artefacts', *Economic and Political Weekly*, July 6–13.

29 Bardhan, P. (1982) 'Little girls and death in India', *Economic and Political Weekly*, 17.

30 Lipton, M. (1977) *Why Poor People Stay Poor: urban bias in developing countries*, Temple Smith and Harvard.

31 World Bank (1989) *India: Poverty, Employment and Social Services*, Country Studies, Washington, DC, World Bank, p. 53.

32 A comparable case is the Irish famine of 1846–7. People died in their tens of thousands, while the food flowed from Ireland to England. That was market success; the market demand was there in England and it was not there in Ireland. The operation was 'successful' in market terms; the patients died only because they could not pay.

33 These data are calculated from Bardhan, P. (1984) *Land, Labour and Rural Poverty*, Oxford. They epitomize the limits of migration as a cure for poverty. Some standard economists would predict that poor labourers will move to the irrigated areas if poverty is less there. In that case, there should be little difference in poverty incidence between these irrigated and dry areas. Also, such an economist will argue, capital will move to the poorer areas, where there are a lot of poor people waiting to work. That does happen but to a surprisingly limited extent – as the persistent regional differences in poverty indicate – even in India, which is a pretty well functioning labour market in many respects. Language, transport costs, risks and the seasonality of labour requirements all limit the scope for migration of labour; as for capital, lenders often prefer local markets that they know well, even if 'cheap labour' could in principle bring higher returns to their lending elsewhere.

34 The proportion of total World Bank lending that went to agricultural projects declined from about one-third in the late 1970s to about one-fifth in 1987–90 (Lipton, M. and Paarlberg, R. (1991) 'Changing missions at the World Bank', *World Policy Journal*, Summer). The proportion of government expenditure by non-oil-producing developing countries that went to agriculture and allied activities fell steadily from 76.9 per cent in 1975 to 4.5 per cent in 1988 (Lipton, M. (1992) 'Accelerated resource degradation by Third World agriculture: created in the commons, in the West, or in bed?', in S. A. Vosti, T. Reardon and W. von Urff (eds) *Agricultural Sustainability, Growth and Poverty Alleviation: issues and policies*, Proceedings of Conference held September 1991, Feldafing, IFPRI/DSE/ZEL, Feldafing.

FURTHER READING

Drèze, J. and Sen, A. K. (1991) *Hunger and Public Action*, Oxford, Clarendon Press.

Lipton, M. with Longhurst, R. (1989) *New Seeds and Poor People*, London, Unwin Hyman.

Sen, A. K. (1981) *Poverty and Famines*, Oxford, Clarendon Press.

World Bank (1990, 1992) *World Development Report 1990* (on poverty) and *World Development Report 1992* (on environment), Washington, DC, World Bank.

9

Food, Old and New: What Limitations?

Ross Buckland

My involvement with the subject of food differs significantly from that of the other contributors to this volume. Since the early 1970s I have been involved in the manufacture, development and marketing of food products: activities aimed at satisfying consumer needs by providing nutritious, high-quality, value-for-money products while at the same time earning a profit. Profit is an essential part of the free enterprise system. It is, however, the 'means', not the 'end'. Profit enables investment in plant and equipment, and in research and development. Shareholders benefit by receipt of dividends, and increases in the value of their shares; employees benefit by increases in earnings and pensions and, importantly at all times, but particularly in recessionary times, by enhanced job security. Lastly, but by no means least, profit enables companies to invest in communities and to discharge their responsibilities as corporate citizens. It is for these reasons that I am totally committed to the company of which I am a part, and to its' achieving consistent, profitable growth.

The world of food marketing is unique and exciting. Compare, for instance, the purchase of a new car; if problems are experienced, the manufacturer/retailer generally has two or more years to eradicate any bad memories. Not so in the food business. The purchaser must be satisfied today. Advertising and price may cause an initial purchase, but without consumer satisfaction with regard to taste, texture, value for money and convenience, then a repeat purchase does not take place in a purchase cycle which is measured not in years, but in days or weeks.

Throughout the centuries we have grown and harvested grain, meat, fish, fruit and vegetables. We have, in many instances, modified these so as to provide higher-yielding and disease-resistant grains and leaner beef, or to preserve fish species and stocks and the ecology of our seas and oceans. We have combined ingredients in different ways to produce new foods and to create and satisfy changing consumer needs.

The energy needs of nineteenth-century workers were far higher than for most of their twentieth-century counterparts. A former colleague of mine who was, and still is, a good and regular squash player, returned from his first medical (at the age of 35) somewhat put out: he had been informed that he was in quite good physical condition for a sedentary, middle-aged executive. Changing energy needs have created opportunities for companies to address specific 'meal occasions', and to assist changes in the eating habits of nations. My former company did not exist at the turn of the twentieth century. Nor did the ready-to-eat breakfast cereal industry. Today my former company alone has sales exceeding US$6 billion annually, and the major Western countries consume more than double that amount each year. Employment has thereby been provided for tens of thousands.

Eating habits have changed and, in countries such as Spain, a new meal occasion has been created. Yet such changes are slow and costly: 'old habits die hard'.

In the dietary construction or reconstruction of a social event such as breakfast, consumer and/or parental education and acceptance is essential. The communication of the attributes of new and different products or food categories is a prerequisite to their trial. The marketing of new products or food categories is expensive, and subject to many potential pitfalls. For instance, in Spain in the early 1980s, 'foreign' products suffered dramatic declines in sales. The shattering of consumer confidence which occurred had nothing to do with the products themselves; rather it was caused by the adulterated olive oil tragedy. This adulteration of a traditional product, sold door-to-door, caused consumers to revert to purchasing brands which they had known for many years, and resulted in the shunning of 'foreign' new products.

Parental education is, in many instances, the key to changing habits. Parents' concern to ensure good nutrition and a balanced diet for their child may not significantly change the eating habits of the parents, but it can, via the child, change the eating habits of a nation.

Changes in the foods we eat have taken place for many different reasons, and some of these will be addressed under the following headings: (1) foods for healthier living; (2) new food additives and ingredients; (3) new food sources; and (4) new food processing technologies.

Foods for Healthier Living

One group of foods for healthier living may be described as 'low in' or 'light' foods. These phrases are used here to denote versions of standard foods that have a lower content of what may be believed to be an undesirable or even harmful component such as calories, fats, sugar and salt. They

Table 9.1 New products introduced in the USA, 1987–9

	Year		
Claim	*1987*	*1988*	*1989*
Reduced/low in:			
Calorie	432	475	962
Fat	159	275	626
Sugar	120	52	188
Salt	281	202	378
Total	992	1004	2154

Source: *Prepared Foods* (1990) Vol. 159, No. 8, p. 48.

are widely available in many product categories and are one of the big growth areas for new products, as shown in table 9.1, which lists new products with 'reduced', 'light' or 'low in' claims introduced in the USA during 1987 to 1989. The area of greatest growth in the UK since the early 1980s has been that of low fat/low saturates. Now widely available are low fat versions of milk, cheese, yoghurt, butter and margarine, together with meat products, salad dressings, frozen meals, frozen desserts and bakery goods.

Reducing the fat content of a food will affect factors such as appearance, texture, flavour, mouthfeel and nutritional value (via the loss of fat-soluble vitamins), and may also affect handling and processing characteristics, storage stability and use in the home. It is easy to produce acceptable low fat versions of some products, with or without the restoration of characteristics of the full fat product, for example skimmed and semi-skimmed milk or low fat milk drinks with added skimmed milk powder and vitamins (to restore mouthfeel and nutritive value). Other products have required much research and development in order to produce acceptable low fat versions, for example low fat spreads, where emulsifiers, stabilizers and thickeners are almost always necessary, and where processing conditions need careful control in order to produce products resembling butter or margarine. The development of fat substitutes will enable low fat foods with better organoleptic characteristics to be made. To some extent, stabilizers and thickeners are already being used as partial fat substitutes.

The changes in milk and low fat spreads can be seen in tables 9.2 and 9.3. Of the low fat milks, skimmed and semi-skimmed had roughly equal market shares until 1986, when the growth of the semi-skimmed share accelerated such that in 1990 it was twice as large as the skimmed milk share. In the

Table 9.2 Market changes in milk in the UK, 1983–91

% sales	*1983*	*1985*	*1987*	*1989*	*1991*
Whole	96.5	86.0	75.0	65.5	56.0
Low fat[a]	3.5	14.0	25.0	34.5	44.0

[a]skimmed and semi-skimmed

Source: National Dairy Council.

Table 9.3 Market changes in spreads in the UK, 1985–90

% sales	*1985*	*1986*	*1987*	*1988*	*1989*	*1990*
Margarine	51	55	55	53	50	48
Butter	39	31	30	28	26	26
Low/reduced fat spreads	10	14	15	19	24	26

Source: National Food Survey.

spreads market, low fat spreads more than doubled their market share between 1985 and 1990.

Low sugar content is another growth area. Unlike fat, sugar has usually to be replaced, at least partially, by alternative sweeteners, as sweetness is not a characteristic that consumers wish to lose. If an intense sweetener is used, then bulking agents must also be added to replace the bulk of the missing sugar. This will, in general, mean additional costs. Most foods that contain sugar can be converted to a low sugar variant. Often foods containing both fat and sugar will be reduced in both so that a low calorie claim can be made.

Salt in food products generally has one or two primary functions: as a preservative, or as a taste enhancer. Either one can be difficult or impossible to substitute. On taste, the final arbiter is neither the scientist nor the manufacturer, but the consumer.

The second group of 'foods for healthier living' are fortified and 'functional' foods. Technological advances in recent decades have enabled not only the restoration of vitamins and minerals lost during processing, but also the fortification of foods to levels nutritionally recommended. 'Functional' foods are foods that may be seen as beneficial in themselves – in practice, there is no clear boundary between functional and other foods, as many so-called functional foods also incorporate perceived 'healthy' ingredients. The Japanese, in particular, have focused on the marketing of foods which have perceived 'functionality', although many products in the UK incorporate fortification or functionality as part of their satisfaction of consumer needs. All food is, or should be, functional, in the sense that it fulfils a purpose and contributes to a healthy diet. What, then, is so special about functional foods? The phenomenon is, we are told, 'the biggest innovation to hit the Japanese food market for a decade and is about to enter the European food market'.[1]

It is estimated that there is now a £1.5 billion market in Japan for food and drink products for which specific physiological claims could be made and that this could grow to £4 billion when appropriate control and monitoring systems have been set up by the Japanese government. At present, more than 70 per cent of these products are soft drinks, but other food sectors include dairy products, confectionery and ready meals. They are not special foods, but are eaten regularly as part of a normal diet. Legislation is currently being prepared in Japan to control and sanction health claims for 12 groups of functional food ingredients, including dietary fibre, minerals, vitamins, unsaturated fatty acids, lactic acid bacteria, oligosaccharides, proteins and peptides. Developments with respect to each of these ingredients are summarized below.

The benefits of insoluble fibre – the reduction of the risk of colon cancer and the elimination of constipation – are well documented.[2] The lowering of blood cholesterol via soluble fibre is also important to health, although an appropriate diet is wellnigh essential to be efficacious. In the United States in 1989, psyllium was added to two bran cereals. Psyllium is a high fibre grain grown mainly in India and contains 80 per cent soluble fibre (as opposed to 10 per cent in oat bran). Until then, psyllium had not been widely used in foods, although for many years in the US it had been an ingredient in certain laxative preparations. This prompted a major US drug company to challenge claims relating psyllium to the lowering of cholesterol on the basis that psyllium should be considered a drug and should not be included in food products without the approval of the Food and Drugs Administration (FDA). A long-drawn-out battle ensued between the two food companies and the regulatory authorities, resulting in one product being withdrawn and the other changing its name and modifying its claims. Such disputes and resolutions are likely to occur again in the future, despite all parties' best efforts to reach agreement on claims regarding efficacy.

It has been recognized for many years that minerals and vitamins are essential to well-being and are today added to food products to supplement those naturally occurring in foodstuffs or to replace those lost during essential processing. Iron and calcium are two key minerals frequently added – the first particularly addressing the needs of women, and the latter responding to concern with respect to osteoporosis. An ongoing area of re-evaluation is that of recommended intake levels, since there is much variation in recommendations from country to country.

Since the late 1960s, margarine and cooking oils with high levels of polyunsaturated fats have been marketed, supported by medical evidence. Medical opinion is now less sure of the positive benefits of large increases in the consumption of polyunsaturated fatty acids (as opposed to decreases in saturated fatty acid consumption). Claims are now being made that increased consumption of monounsaturated fatty acids and of essential fatty acids (long-chain polyunsaturated or 4 omega-3 fatty acids) would be equally or more beneficial. Fish-oil supplements have been available in the UK for several years, but their consumption is minimal. In the early 1990s, a high monounsaturated fatty acid spread was launched.

With regard to lactic acid bacteria, the food industry's focus has moved from their use in cultured dairy products, such as yoghurt, to specific bacteria such as *Bifidobacterium* species and *Lactobacillus acidophilus*, which are normal inhabitants of the human large intestine. These bacteria have been used in products promoted in Germany for over 30 years ('Bioghurt', 'Biogarde'), and have become popular in France, where they account for over 10 per cent of the yoghurt market. They are relatively new to the UK market, accounting for only 1 per cent of yoghurts. Products such as butter, sour cream, fresh cheese and hard cheese containing *Bifidobacteria* and *Lactobacillus acidophilus* are also available in Continental Europe.

In Japan, other lactic acid bacteria are also promoted. In Eastern Europe and the former USSR, products containing lactic acid bacteria and yeasts (kefir, koumiss) are popular and are regarded as having health benefits. The claimed benefits of lactic acid bacteria are: the prevention of constipation; the inhibition of harmful bacteria in the gut; the promotion of the immune system; and less production of toxic substances in the large intestine. A major doubt about dietary lactic acid bacteria is whether a large enough proportion of the intake (1) survives transit through the stomach and small intestine, and (2) establishes itself in the large intestine – such questions need to be resolved in order for appropriate product development to occur.

Oligosaccharides are a group of sugars made up of small chains of one or more simple sugars (such as glucose or fructose) and are found in many food materials derived from natural plants. The best-know example of an oligosaccharide is common sugar-sucrose (consisting of one unit of glucose plus one unit of fructose). It is claimed that certain oligosaccharides consisting of several fructose units encourage the survival and growth of *bifidus* and *acidophilus* bacteria in the human gut. As explained above, the presence of these bacteria in the gut is claimed to aid digestion, to promote the functioning of the immune system and to dissolve gut carcinogens. Fruit juice products fortified with oligosaccharides are already on sale in Japan.

Otsuka Pharmaceutical makes Japan's best-selling soft drink, called 'Fibemini', which the manufacturers claim contains all the minerals, vitamins and fibre the body needs in a day. Japanese 'stamina drinks' have become hugely popular, with more than 200 brands available. The products come in small bottles and are taken for added punch to relieve hangovers; manufacturers of the most expensive brands even claim that the drinks improve sexual performance. However, according to an article published in the US medical journal *Archives of Medicine*, coffee is a cheaper alternative![3]

It is well known that protein is an essential part of the diet. The breakdown products from protein (peptides) usually take the form of small protein chains of lower molecular weights which makes them more rapidly absorbed. Indeed, this is one of the reasons for the established use of peptides in enteral feeding products. Researchers in Japan have developed a milk protein derivative by treating casein with proteolytic enzymes to produce casein phosphopeptides, which are claimed to increase the absorption of calcium, iron and other minerals and to prevent calcium loss from bones. This compound is already being used in baby milk products in Japan. Of course, many of these so-called functional foods have long been recognized as nutritionally significant; it is important to remember that similar developments have been under way in Western Europe and the USA for a number of years under the banner heading of 'healthy foods'. The underlying difference is that, while functional/healthy claims in Western Europe and the USA have centred on the inclusion of a few comparatively simple ingredients, for example oat bran and *bifidus* bacteria, the Japanese are claiming perceived medical benefits for a wider, more complex range of materials. However, it is important to realize that, until legislation is passed, no products can be designated as functional foods or claim specific medical benefits. In Japan the government is working together with the medical experts to allow specific health claims to be made.[4]

The United States is lagging behind Japan, but is well ahead of Europe in drafting legislation in this area. Whilst proposing legislation which will prohibit unsubstantiated claims, the US Food and Drugs Administration recognizes the principle of linking health claims with specific ingredients and endorses the fundamental premise of functional foods. In sharp contrast, the European Commission (EC) seems to be rigidly opposed to any health claims on foods, even though governments are increasingly recognizing the connection between diet and health. Obviously, it is important that claims can and must be substantiated, but it is naive to believe that a complete ban on all claims will prevent the consumer from being misled by fanciful ideas that have little or no foundation. The absence of information about the nature of a product inhibits consumers' opportunities for informed choice. If food companies are prevented from communicating the positive health benefits of their products to the buying public, then this will stifle innovation, some products may never be brought to market, and the industry's funding of essential research and development projects would, in all likelihood, decline dramatically.

Table 9.4 Alternative sweeteners

Caloric sweeteners
Glucose syrup
High fructose corn syrup
Crystalline fructose
Reduced calorie bulk sweeteners
Sorbitol
Mannitol
Isomalt
Hydrogenated glucose syrup
Xylitol
Artificial intense sweeteners
Saccharin
Aspartame
Acesulfam-K
Cyclamate
Natural intense sweeteners
Thaumatin
Neohesperidin dihydrochalcone

New Food Additives and Ingredients

These can be addressed under the headings of intense sweeteners, fat substitutes and natural additives.

Sweetness is a very desirable taste property in foods, but in the form of sugars it also provides calories. Excessive sugar consumption has been linked to obesity and dental caries and, of course, intake of sugars must be closely monitored by diabetics for health reasons. This has resulted in the development of a range of alternative sweeteners to sugars which can be divided into four types: (1) caloric sweeteners; (2) reduced calorie bulk sweeteners; (3) artificial intense sweeteners; and (4) natural intense sweeteners.

Alternative caloric sweeteners include glucose syrup, high fructose corn syrup and crystalline fructose. High fructose corn syrup is made by enzymic treatment of corn starch and is a mixture of fructose and glucose. The calorific value of sucrose and fructose is the same: 3.75 Kcals/g. However, fructose is 1.3–1.8 times sweeter than sucrose on a weight-for-weight basis. Therefore, a given amount of sucrose can be replaced by a smaller amount of fructose (plus an inert bulking agent) to give a food with a reduced calorie content. Glucose syrup and most high fructose syrups have a sweetness roughly equivalent to that of sucrose. High fructose syrup is now about

30 per cent cheaper than sucrose in the USA and it has almost totally replaced sucrose in soft drinks manufacture. It is also used in foods such as bakery products and ice cream. Crystalline fructose is sweeter than sugar and can be used to produce reduced calorie versions of high sugar content foods.

Reduced calorie bulk sweeteners are sugar alcohols (or polyols) and are very similar in chemical structure to sugars. They are mostly non-metabolized in the small intestine, but may be fermented by bacteria in the large intestine. This means that they are suitable for diabetics, but their excessive intake can lead to gastrointestinal upset. They are all non-cariogenic and generally are less sweet than sucrose. Most are synthesized chemically and all are more expensive than sucrose. UK-approved sugar alcohols are sorbitol, mannitol, isomalt, hydrogenated glucose syrup and xylitol. Sorbitol, mannitol and xylitol all occur naturally but only mannitol can be extracted (from seaweed) in large enough quantities for commercial use. Xylitol has a high cooling sensation in the mouth, which limits its use to certain types of confectionery, for example chewing gum and mints.

Some intense sweeteners are synthesized compounds with a relative sweetness of between 100–1000 times that of sucrose. All are non-caloric in that they are either non-metabolizable or, if metabolized, they contribute insignificant amounts of calories since they are used at such low concentrations. UK-approved intense sweeteners are saccharin, aspartame and Acesulfam-K. Cyclamate is currently banned in the UK but is likely to be approved in a forthcoming EC Directive.

The most widely used intense sweetener, aspartame, was accidentally discovered by a G. D. Searle research worker in 1965, and took 16 years to gain approval by the US government's Food and Drugs Administration, with over 100 trials for safety in use. The US patent expired in 1992, which means that a number of companies are now free to manufacture it.

Aspartame is a dipeptide sweetener which is metabolized by the body to phenylalanine, which can cause problems for the small group of people suffering from phenylketonuria. Phenylketonuria is an inherited metabolic disorder, in which sufferers cannot metabolize phenylalanine, an amino acid found in all proteins, and one of the two amino acids that make up aspartame. Phenylketonurics have to follow a diet of foods that are naturally low in phenylalanine or that have been treated to reduce the phenylalanine content. Aspartame is widely used in 'diet' soft drinks and has been the focus of media attention, despite the extensive research and its approval worldwide by regulatory bodies. Many more intense sweeteners are under development, mostly sugar- or amino acid-based.

The final category of alternative sugars are the so-called natural intense sweeteners, which are derived from natural sources. These include thaumatin extracted from the fruit of a West African plant and neohesperidin dihydrochalcone, derived from a bitter-tasting compound from the peel of Seville oranges.

The main challenge to food industry scientists associated with the use of sweeteners lies in the replacement of sucrose in a product formulation by a sweetener with a different sweetness level. If an intense sweetener is used, then, as mentioned above, a bulking agent must be used to replace the sugar mass. This can lead to increased costs and possible loss of functional properties. The ideal sweetener should have the following properties: the sweetness profile of sucrose; no after-taste; the ability to function and metabolize like sucrose; low or non-existent calorie content; the ability to process easily; and affordability. Unfortunately, the ideal sweetener does not yet exist; the closest match is currently achieved by a combination of sweeteners. The use of intense sweeteners has allowed the development of a whole range of new low calorie products.

Moving on to fat substitutes, fat is the most concentrated source of food energy, providing more than twice the calories on a weight-for-weight basis to that obtained from protein or carbohydrate. In addition, fats contribute to the structure, texture and taste of foods and provide a carrier for fat-soluble vitamins A, D and E. However, studies on the relationship between diet and health have identified the need to moderate fat consumption (in particular the level of saturated fats in the diet) and have increased consumer awareness of the need for a healthy diet.

This awareness has created a demand for low calorie or calorie-reduced foods which in turn has stimulated the development of a wide range of fat substitutes with little or no calorific value. In terms of composition, fat substitutes can be divided into four main categories: (1) emulsifiers and stabilizers; (2) carbohydrate-based fat substitutes; (3) protein-based fat substitutes; and (4) synthetic materials.

The use of permitted thickeners and stabilizers, for example xanthan gum in products such as ice cream and salad dressings, can reproduce the viscosity and mouthfeel of the original product, but it is difficult to achieve much more than a 50 per cent reduction in fat content without loss of texture. In the same way, permitted emulsifiers such as polyglycerol esters of fatty acids can be used to stabilize low fat versions of conventional emulsion-based foods such as ice cream, margarine, confectionery coatings and bakery products.

A number of carbohydrate-based products are available, derived from hydrolysed starches (dextrins and maltodextrins) obtained from natural sources such as rice, tapioca, corn or potato. These materials are often used as concentrated aqueous solutions which can replace fat on a 1:1 basis, cutting calorific values by up to 75 per cent. Applications include low fat spreads, salad dressings, dips and frozen desserts. These products have been in use in the United States since the early 1980s and meet the Food and Drug Administration's 'generally recognized as safe' (GRAS) requirements as they are based on natural food ingredients.

Similarly, in recent years a range of protein-based products derived from egg and whey protein sources has emerged. The first product on the market and the best-known example in this category is 'Simplesse', marketed by the Nutrasweet Company. It is produced by a microparticulation process which involves heat treatment to coagulate the protein, followed by a high shear process to form very small uniform particles of less than 3 micron in size which create the same mouthfeel characteristics as fat. 'Simplesse' has been 'generally recognized as safe' by the FDA for use in mayonnaise and frozen dairy desserts, and has recently found a much wider application in salad dressings, ice cream, low fat spreads and yoghurt. In 1992, a major retailer in the UK launched a 5 per cent fat spread and a bioyoghurt containing 'Simplesse'. Unfortunately, protein-based substitutes are adversely affected by heat which somewhat limits their use in processed foods.

The fourth category of fat substitutes are the synthetic products which are fatty in nature and which can withstand high temperatures, qualities which make them suitable for use in frying oils and heat-processed foods. These products are not metabolized and therefore do not contribute any calories to the food. In theory, they can replace fat totally with little effect on the organoleptic properties of a food, but in practice they are likely to be used at levels of between 35–75 per cent.

Unfortunately, no synthetic fat substitute has as yet received regulatory approval. Olestra, developed by Proctor & Gamble, is the best-known synthetic fat analogue. It was first discovered in 1968 and has been under continual development ever since. Chemically, it is a sucrose polyester, that is, a molecule of sucrose esterified with six, seven or eight fatty acid entities. Production methods and uses have been widely patented by Proctor & Gamble. A petition for FDA approval for its use in cooking oil and fried snack products was filed in 1987, but as yet has not been approved. Objections from consumer bodies in the USA to its approval have centred on the adequacy of the toxicological studies.

The move towards natural additives has grown as part of a reaction against anything artificial, and the consequent trend has been towards the use of natural-additive and preservative-free foods only. The natural versus artificial debate is based on the unjustified belief that natural foods and/or natural additives are inherently safer than processed foods and artificial additives. Foods without additives are not necessarily safer since the major threat to food safety is microbiological rather than toxicological. The number of cases of food poisoning due to pathogenic micro-organisms far exceeds the number of cases of toxic poisoning due to chemical additives or even naturally occurring contaminants. With the move towards convenience foods and fewer shopping occasions, the removal of preservatives from food can result in early spoilage or the growth of undesirable micro-organisms which may cause food poisoning if storage conditions are not carefully observed.

Several modern food products could not exist without the use of emulsifiers or stabilizers. All additives, both natural and artificial, have to undergo strict testing to prove that they are safe at the highest possible usage levels. A small number of natural additives, as well as artificial additives, have had approval withdrawn for safety reasons, often because experimental data to satisfy the present criteria were unavailable, and their commercial value did not justify additional expenditure on tests. It is estimated that the cost of securing clearance today for a new additive exceeds £1/2 million.

Likewise, natural and 'nature-identical' colours are taking a growing share of the market. The number of artificial colours approved for UK food use has fallen over the last two decades whilst new natural colours have been added to the approved list. Natural colours are mainly plant extracts, for example curcumin, chlorophylls, carotenes and beetroot red. Some of the carotenes and riboflavins (nature-identical) have the added bonus of being vitamins or vitamin precursors.

Some artificial antioxidants do have question marks over their safety, but the shift to natural antioxidants is at an early stage. Ascorbic acid (vitamin C) and tocopherols (vitamin E) are the major natural antioxidants. Another research area which several US companies are investigating is the use of rosemary extracts. Applications include meat and poultry products, salad dressings, snacks, nuts and fats and oils. Several approved preservatives are found in natural sources in very small amounts, for example sorbic, benzoic and propionic acids. The major research area for natural preservatives is likely to be microbial cultures, especially lactic cultures, for example 'alta', 'microgard' and 'lysolac', all of which are claimed to extend the shelf life of food by inhibiting the growth of spoilage organisms.

New Food Sources

Modern biotechnology can be used to provide new sources of foods and food ingredients or to improve the characteristics or productivity of current sources of food.

Biotechnology encompasses a range of biological techniques, including genetic engineering, enzyme technology, fermentation and plant cell cultures. Some of these techniques are new, others are very old and have been used in food production for a long time. Brewing, wine-making, cheese-making and vinegar manufacture are all biotechnological methods of food production. Genetic engineering is the direct alteration of the genetic complement of an organism by deleting a gene or inserting a gene from another source. Plant cell culture and genetic engineering can be used to achieve the same results as conventional breeding, but at a much faster rate, or can be used to achieve results that would be impossible using conventional breeding techniques.

Biotechnology and New Food Sources

Microbial proteins have had a chequered history. In the 1970s, the production of protein by growing yeasts and bacteria on hydrocarbons (alkanes, natural gas) and carbohydrates (whey, agricultural wastes) was seen as an important technology for the future. Many large projects were proposed; some were built, a few reached commercial production (BP's 'toprina', ICI's 'pruteen') and all have now closed. Rising oil prices caused most to become uneconomic, though small-scale yeast production on whey was not affected and has continued in operation. Because of concerns about safety, most hydrocarbon-based projects were for feedstuffs, though the original intention was to produce foods by this technology. Large-scale feedstuffs production reportedly only occurred in the former USSR. One product that was developed over a long period of time (20 years) and was successfully commercialized is 'Quorn'.

'Quorn' is a fibrous product (mycoprotein) derived from a strain of *Fusarium* mould, grown in a glucose solution obtained by hydrolysis of wheat starch. Originally developed by Rank Hovis McDougall (RHM), it is now made by Marlow Foods, a joint venture of RHM and ICI, incorporating ICI's technology. The mould (or microfungus) is continuously harvested, heat-shocked to halt growth and reduce nucleic acid levels, and dried to form sheets of mycoprotein. The filamentous structure of mycoprotein gives it great similarity to the fibrous structure of meat, and the further processing of mycoprotein into 'Quorn' is aimed at enhancing its meat-like properties.

A major retailer launched the first retail product containing 'Quorn' in 1985, and the range of branded and own-label foods containing it has grown steadily. 'Quorn' itself was launched as a retail product in 1989.

Several food ingredients have been commercially produced by fermentation technology for some time. Examples are food acids such as citric and lactic, and food enzymes such as proteases, lipases, lactase and mould-derived rennet substitutes.

A more recent example, using genetic engineering, is the production of chymosin, the active enzyme of calf rennet. The gene for chymosin production has been transferred from calf stomach cells to bacteria, which produce the enzyme when grown in a fermenter. The use of this enzyme, now officially approved, overcomes the shortage of calf rennet without recourse to the use of rennet substitutes, which have not been found to be 100 per cent satisfactory. The enzyme chymosin is produced in the fourth stomach of calves, but not of adult cattle. Calf rennet is in short supply because the growth of cheese production has not been matched by growth in the number of calves slaughtered. Rennet substitutes, which are different enzymes produced from a variety of animal, microbial and plant sources, do not have the same enzyme action. The balance of milk-clotting activity to proteolytic activity varies, giving differences in the quality and yield of cheese.

The optimization of cheese starter cultures is also under investigation. Many desirable metabolic functions of starter cultures are linked to genes carried in plasmid DNA, not DNA in the nucleus. This means they are unstable, since the plasmids, and therefore the functions, can be lost during starter multiplication. Genetic engineering allows the possibility of maximizing and stabilizing these desirable functions and also of constructing strains that would accelerate cheese ripening by premature starter death and release of intracellular enzymes.

A key element of the EC Food Law Harmonization Programme is to establish a procedure for the evolution and approval of such new foods and ingredients in order to ensure consumer safety and to promote consumer confidence.

New Food Processing Technologies

For many years conventional pasteurization and sterilization techniques have been successfully used by the food industry and these processing methods have established an excellent track record for producing high-quality safe products.

Since the late 1980s, a number of new processing technologies have emerged which are designed to extend the shelf life of aseptically processed high-quality foods containing particulate materials for both chilled and ambient storage.

The rapid growth of the chilled recipe dish market in France in the mid-1980s saw the widespread introduction of the use of a little-known technology called 'sous-vide' processing which had previously been used primarily as a catering technique for the production of very short shelf life recipe dishes. It consists of the preparation and, if necessary, the partial pre-cooking of food, using a gentle heat treatment process at temperatures below 65°C followed by rapid cooling and vacuum-packing into plastic bags or pouches which are then stored under chill conditions and reheated before consumption. This type of cook-chill process can present some risks as cooking at very low temperatures does not destroy heat-resistant spores of organisms such as *Clostridium botulinum* which can then subsequently grow to form toxins if the pack is subjected to temperature abuse. This prompted the UK government to issue a warning statement in 1989 and to propose much tighter controls on food processes involving vacuum-packing.

Nevertheless, the French market for 'sous-vide' type products in consumer packs has seen rapid growth since its inception in 1986. These products are claimed to be of the same high quality as freshly cooked meals with shelf lives of between 21–42 days when stored under refrigerated conditions.

Conventional in-can sterilization techniques enable food to be stored at ambient temperatures for long periods, in excess of six months. However, the quality may be poor because of the need for high-temperature peripheral heating to ensure effective heat transfer to the centre of the container to effect a *botulinum* kill. This is especially so with large cans which are used for catering purposes.

Aseptic processing of food using plate, tubular or scraped surface heat exchangers, followed by aseptic filling into paperboard or plastic containers, has been used by the milk industry for over 30 years. Unfortunately, this method does not lend itself easily to products containing large particulates such as chunks of meat, vegetables or fruit.

A recent advance is the application of Ohmic heating, which involves passing an electrical current through a continuous flow of food product. The electrical resistance of the food causes heat to be generated, which sterilizes the product within a matter of minutes. Heat penetration through the product is far more even and rapid, resulting in high levels of flavour retention and particulate integrity. Ohmic heating is now being used commercially for the production of high-quality recipe dishes matching cook-chill products, but with the added benefit of safe long-term storage under ambient conditions. The Ohmic heating process has been approved by the Government Advisory Committee on Novel Foods and Processes (ACNFP) for the production of shelf-stable ready meals.

Another method for extending the shelf life of food ingredients and products is irradiation. The technique was developed in the early part of the twentieth century and over the last four decades, food irradiation has probably been studied more than any other food preservation process. The results of the research have been considered by independent national and international expert scientific committees, including the UK's Advisory Committee on Irradiated and Novel Foods (ACINF), the World Health Organization (WHO), the Food and Agriculture Organization's Joint Expert Committee on Food Irradiation and the EC Scientific Committee for Food. All have concluded that food irradiation is a safe process.

Irradiation of food has been shown to be effective in destroying pathogenic micro-organisms such as salmonella, listeria and campylobacter. It has proved its value as a treatment for poultry and meat and some shellfish. For certain produce, such as dried herbs and spices, irradiation can be used to destroy insects, pests and bacterial contamination, in place of chemical fumigation methods which are subject to concern on health grounds. For example, ethylene oxide, which was used for this purpose, is banned in EC countries and is no longer permitted in the UK. However, irradiation is not suitable for use on all foods. Some fruits, for example, are softened by irradiation and some fatty foods develop a rancid flavour.

The irradiation of food has been approved for use in some countries for over 20 years and is currently used in 21 countries, including Belgium, France, the Netherlands and the United States. In the UK, irradiation has been used for over 30 years to sterilize medical equipment, certain pharmaceuticals, cosmetics and packaging.

In 1991 the UK government announced its intention to permit the use of irradiation as a legal means of preserving food. Regulations on the control of irradiation plants and the labelling of irradiated food were introduced at the same time. However, despite government reassurance, many consumers remain unconvinced about the safety and efficacy of food irradiation. Many have doubts about the process on the grounds that it provides yet another example of 'scientists' interfering with the nation's food supply'. Some of this concern and doubt is attributable to the term 'irradiation' itself, especially in the wake of the Chernobyl nuclear power station accident. Despite the fact that ionizing irradiation does not make food radioactive, it is hard to convince people of this fact. Most major food retailers have said they will not stock irradiated foods, others say they may stock it if there is sufficient demand. Food manufacturers will be extremely cautious before they decide to use the irradiation process. For example, the irradiation of herbs and spices was thought to be an obvious application following the banning of ethylene oxide sterilization, but manufacturers have bypassed it by developing new processes based on extrusion or steam sterilization.

A very recent and interesting development which is attracting considerable attention is the application of high-pressure sterilization to preserve food without heat and hence improve the quality by reducing heat damage. High-pressure effects on food can be produced by applying hydrostatic pressures ranging from 1000–10 000 kg/sqcm. Research work in Japan has demonstrated the effectiveness of this process in destroying microorganisms in various foods, accompanied by beneficial flavour and texture changes in meat, fish and egg products.

In conclusion, it is essential to have a recognition of the importance of research and the opportunities which the results of that research can provide. From a commercial standpoint, it is therefore critical that those involved in research and changing scientific knowledge liaise closely with their counterparts in marketing, production and senior management to ensure that existing products, where appropriate, are modified and the right new products are launched.

NOTES

1 *Food Manufacture* (1991) Vol. 66, No. 1, p. 26.

2 Trowell, H., Burkitt, D. and Heaton, K. (1985) *Dietary Fibre, Fibre-Depleted Foods and Disease*, London, Academic Press.

3 *Food Manufacture* (1991) Vol. 66, No. 1, p. 27.
4 P. A. Consulting Group (1990) *Functional Foods: a new global added value market?*, London, PA Consulting Group.

FURTHER READING

Foods for healthier living

'"Low and light" foods and drinks – meeting consumer demand', Leatherhead Food R.A. Symposium Proceedings No. 48, 1990.

P.A. Consulting Group (1990) *Functional Foods: a new global added value market?*, London, P.A. Consulting Group.

International Dairy Federation (1983) 'Cultured dairy foods in human nutrition', International Dairy Federation Bulletin No. 159.

New food additives and ingredients

Nabors, L. O'B. and Gelardi, R. C. (1986) *Alternative Sweeteners*, New York, Marcel Dekker.

Lee, S. (1991) *Fat Substitutes – an update*, Leatherhead Food R.A. Food Focus No. 15.

10

The International Relations of Food: The Unfolding Crisis of National Regulation

Harriet Friedmann

Introduction

International conflict over agricultural regulation long dominated the Uruguay Round of the General Agreement on Tariffs and Trade (GATT), threatening agreements that greatly extend corporate power relative to national (and public) power. At issue, paradoxically, was a type of national regulation of agriculture whose days were numbered. Even more paradoxically, Europe, cast as defender of the old ways, committed itself to more basic domestic reform than the United States. Major changes were initiated in the European Common Agricultural Policy which went further than anyone imagined possible at the outset of the Uruguay Round.[1] The choice in 1994 is not between 'regulation' or 'free trade', therefore, but between new forms of regulation.

In and around the tangled web of national politics, European and North American integration and international economic competition, new protagonists are emerging. The contest over new rules and relations for food and agriculture also depends on transnational corporations (TNCs) and on popular movements, neither of which are formally present at the negotiations.

This chapter was originally presented as a paper at Wolfson College, Oxford, and revised versions at the Agrarian Studies Program, Yale University, and the Department of Political Science, University of Toronto, and benefited from discussion with participants. I would like to thank Henry Bernstein, Barbara Harriss-White, Geoffrey Kay, Jean Laux, Philip McMichael and Mary Summers for critical advice and encouragement in revising earlier drafts, and Yildiz Atasoy for invaluable research assistance.

Agricultural support programmes were put in place roughly half a century ago in response to farm politics. Since then, farms have become suppliers of raw materials within a transnational agro-food sector dominated by some of the largest, most technically dynamic corporations in the world. At the same time, urbanization and the rise of social movements expressing interests of consumers, environmentalists and others, have shifted the political focus away from farm incomes.

In the long view, it is clear that the agricultural trade conflicts inside and outside the GATT were the culmination of changes in the international political economy. The rules implicitly governing agro-food relations had been created in the years immediately after World War II and worked stably enough for nearly 25 years to justify the idea of a 'food regime'. However, new economic alignments developed during that time, which by the early 1970s began to undermine the international relations of food.

In this chapter, I analyse the rise of a food regime and the emergence of contradictory and conflictual relations within it. First, I define the food regime and its main features. In the second section, I describe the character of the food regime, including its internal tensions, between 1947 and 1973. In the third section, I describe the emergence of new relations and new rules after the food crisis of 1972–73. To simplify the story of the regime and its crisis, in these sections I treat states, particularly the US, as integral actors.[2] In the final part of this chapter, I explore the residual and emergent relations which make possible either new regimes, or the descent into deeper disorder.

The Food Regime: Principles and Contradictions

The impasse in international economic relations has centred on agriculture because in the agro-food sector there exists the largest gap between national regulation and transnational economic organization. This gap is the legacy of the post-World War II food regime, the rule-governed structure of production and consumption of food on a world scale. The food regime was created in 1947 when alternative international regulation in the form of the proposal for a World Food Board was rejected.[3] At the GATT, the only clear positions were those which 'decouple' and 'deregulate' elements of a food regime that no longer works. The present alternatives for a new regime are not formally proposed. They must be teased out from analyses of the social forces involved in global agro-food restructuring.

The post-war food regime was governed by informal rules, which nonetheless had the capacity to regulate property and power within and between nations. The food regime, therefore, was partly about international relations of food, and partly about the world food economy. The regulation of the food regime both underpinned and reflected the balances of power among states, organized national lobbies, classes – farmers, workers, peasants – and capital. The implicit rules evolved through practical experiences and negotiations among states, ministries, corporations, farm lobbies, consumer lobbies and others, in response to immediate problems of production, distribution and trade. Out of this web of practices emerged a stable pattern of production and power that lasted for two and a half decades.

The rules defining the food regime gave priority to national regulation, and authorized both import controls and export subsidies necessary to manage national farm programmes. These national programmes, particularly at the outset the United States' New Deal commodity programmes, generated chronic surpluses. As these played out, they structured a specific set of international relations in which power – to restructure international trade and production in one state's favour – was wielded in the unusual form of subsidized exports of surplus commodities. In this way agriculture, which was always central to the world economy, was an exceptional international sector.

Then, the 'food crisis' of the early 1970s, combined with simultaneous money and oil crises, initiated a period of instability from which we have not yet recovered. The sense of crisis in the early 1970s stemmed from the sudden, unexpected shift from surplus to scarcity, which sent grain prices soaring and threatened food shortages for poor people and most of all, for poor countries. In retrospect, it is clear that since the shortages came from a one-time explosion of demand and a temporary drop in production, the basic cause of surpluses was bound to reassert itself. Since major states continued to support agricultural prices by purchasing commodities, within a few years farmers produced more surpluses, and states resumed mercantile trade practices to get rid of them.

With the reappearance of surpluses, old policies designed to deal with them once again seemed appropriate, and problems with those policies were not regarded as being connected to the trajectory of international food relations since 1947.[4] However, the disappearance of the symptom simply masked the survival of the disorder. New relations which had emerged within the regime became significant enough to alter the pattern. Old practices, especially surplus disposal in foreign markets, could not reconstruct the original relations of power and property. Food aid or other forms of export subsidy, which once underpinned the food regime, came instead to express intense international conflicts.

The Surplus Regime, 1947–1972

Because the US protected its own domestic markets, other countries were constrained to adopt similar agricultural policies focused on the national market. US trade restrictions, designed to protect domestic farm programmes, encouraged other states to focus on their own national agro-food sectors. States replicated the US regulation of national sectors, but adapted policies to their locations in the food regime. For Continental Europe, this meant shifting the focus of protective agricultural policies away from tariffs, and redesigning trade protection around domestic support for farm prices. For other parts of the world, adaptation of the US model involved parallel shifts in the forms of state agricultural regulation. Thus, the post-war rules did not liberalize national agricultural policy, but created a new pattern of intensely national regulation.

At the same time, the free movement of investment capital tended to integrate the agro-food sectors of Europe and the US into an Atlantic agro-food economy. This tension framed the new roles of tropical export countries, including former European colonies, in the food regime. This integration, moreover, was uneven. It did not include the countries of the socialist bloc, and, despite high levels of aid and trade, the capitalist countries of Asia were not integrated into transnational agro-food complexes.

Thus the post-war food regime was built on a tension between the replication and the integration of national agro-food sectors. The tension between replication and integration reflected on an international scale the problem inherent in US farm programmes – chronic surpluses.

The United States at the Centre

Paradoxically, the main challenge to present rules comes from the source of those same rules in the early post-war years – the US state. New Deal farm programmes of the 1930s were retained after World War II, despite widespread awareness of the problem of surpluses. Mercantile practices had to be used to dispose of the surpluses and to prevent a flood of imports into the US. As the dominant economic power after World War II, the US insisted on international rules consistent with its own national farm support programmes. These rules eventually allowed the US to create an overwhelming preponderance in world agro-food production and trade, far beyond its historic share.[5]

Yet mercantilist agricultural policy was in conflict with the larger US policy to promote free movement of goods and money internationally.[6] Because of its weight in creating international institutions after World War II, US decisions transferred this tension to the food regime as a whole.

The food regime was created by a series of decisions between 1945 and 1949, which reflected US determination to protect the import controls and export subsidies which, as we shall see, were a necessary complement to its domestic farm policy. US commitment to mercantile agricultural trade practices led to the sacrifice of multilateral institutions which had wide support among post-war governments, not only for regulating food, but also for the pursuit of the larger US agenda for liberal trade. The World Food Board Proposal, which provided for global supply management and food aid through the Food and Agriculture Organization (FAO), was rejected by the US and Britain at an international conference in Washington, DC in 1947. The Havana Treaty creating an International Trade Organization (ITO), a 1946 initiative by the US Department of State, was never formally submitted to Congress because it contradicted mercantile clauses in US domestic farm laws. Even the GATT, which began as an ad hoc negotiating forum intended to be subsumed under the formal powers of the anticipated ITO, and continued as a feeble substitute in its absence, excluded agriculture from its ban on import controls and export subsidies, at US insistence.[7]

The need for trade controls stemmed from an odd feature of domestic farm programmes, where, instead of direct income support, New Deal price supports tried to raise farm incomes indirectly by setting a minimum price for commodities named in the legislation, and maintaining this price through state purchases. Government purchases to support prices encouraged farmers to produce as much as possible. Legislation to limit production by restricting acreage was never effective. In fact, insofar as they encouraged farmers to remove their worst land from production, acreage controls tended to increase productivity.

Surpluses mounted more persistently with the technological developments involved in the industrialization of agriculture. Industrialization subordinated farms to emerging agro-food corporations, both as buyers of machines, chemicals and animal feeds, and as sellers of raw materials to food manufacturing industries or livestock operations. Profits in the agro-food sector depended on the larger restructuring of the post-war economy towards mass production and mass consumption,[8] especially increased consumption of animal products and high value-added manufactured foods, or what might be called 'durable foods'.[9]

Commodity price support programmes both protected family farms and encouraged their relations with agro-food corporations. By supporting prices, the legislation rewarded large family farms. Farms increased productivity and scale through technologies bought from key vehicle and chemical industries. As they became locked onto a technical treadmill, they also became increasingly specialized. The most important shift was the separation of intensive livestock from cereal production, and with it the growth of the two most important crops of the 'second agricultural revolution', hybrid maize and soy. Capital-intensive manufacture of soy-maize animal feeds allowed corporations to place themselves between increasingly specialized intensive livestock operations, which were their customers, and maize and soy farms, which sold to them.[10] At the same time, mass production of durable foods required standard agricultural raw materials, which corporations obtained through contracts with increasingly specialized and standardized farms.[11] As durable foods came to be made from generic ingredients, such as sweeteners, fats and starches, corporations were able to reduce their dependence on specific products and increase the possibilities for substitution.[12]

The key to the persistence of the world food regime was the innovative US policy of foreign aid, combined with import controls. Domestic agricultural price supports required import controls and export subsidies. Without controls, high domestic support prices would attract imports. Apart from its negative impact on hungry people abroad, especially war-torn Europe, this meant that without import controls, the Commodity Credit Corporation, a US government agency, would have to buy ever greater quantities of world supplies to maintain the incomes of US farmers. Moreover, the more it bought, the greater was the gap between support prices and residual 'market' prices. Government stocks put a downward pressure on prices by keeping supply (or potential supply) high. This created fiscal problems for the state budget, which had to pay support prices plus storage and disposal costs. Since the destruction of surplus agricultural products was politically unacceptable in a hungry nation (and world), commodity price support programmes required a way to dispose of surpluses without lowering prices, that is, outside 'markets'. These were found through domestic public distribution, such as food stamps and school lunches, and through subsidized exports to other countries in the form of 'aid'.

Aid allowed the US to turn the problem of surplus stocks into an opportunity to pursue strategic, welfare and economic policies. Yet aid did not simply integrate donor and recipient. As a mercantile trade practice, aid encouraged recipients and competitors alike to adopt the national regulation of agriculture and trade. Thus replication was built into the international food economy at the same time.

In other words, what is frequently called the 'export of the US model' of both production and consumption,[13] was the outcome of specific practices in the post-war food regime. At the same time, these practices also reflected historical experiences, so that the effects were quite distinct in Europe, the emergent Third World and, as we shall see later in the chapter, in Japan. In Europe and the Third World, new links with the US revolved around trade in wheat, animal feeds and raw materials for food manufacturing.

Post-war Europe and the Atlantic Pivot

Marshall aid to Europe simultaneously established the basis for Atlantic agro-food relations, and invented the specific mechanisms of foreign aid which were later adapted to the Third World. For post-war European agriculture, the tension between national regulation, with attendant surpluses, and liberal trade, was reflected in Marshall aid and later in the Common Agricultural Policy. The US supported the European protection of wheat and dairy products, even at the very high level needed to keep out efficiently produced and subsidized US exports. In return, the European Community (EC) exempted maize and soy from the import controls of the Common Agricultural Policy.[14]

Under the Marshall administration, dumping was secondary to recovery. US legislation required the use of Marshall funds to buy US surplus commodities at specified rates as much as 50 per cent below the domestic price; it balanced the contradictory interests of reconstruction and dumping by specifying maximum and minimum quantities to be disposed of in recipient countries. US Marshall administrators, however, minimized agricultural dumping, as they understood it to be.[15] The 40 per cent of Marshall aid that went to food and agriculture in Europe was concentrated upon imports of feedstuffs and fertilizers for agricultural reconstruction. The balance shifted after 1954, when surpluses were redirected to underdeveloped countries in the form of food aid.[16]

However, as soon as agricultural reconstruction showed some success, West European farmers sought US markets for their dairy products. Congress then imposed import quotas on dairy (and a whole range of other) products. This, despite the fact that even with high support prices, imports of dairy products accounted for less than 1 per cent of the US market. The ability of special interests to override US interests in trade relations with Europe can only be understood in the ideological context of the Cold War. The farm lobby got its import restrictions not through agricultural legislation but through an amendment in the Defense Production Act of 1950. In 1952, the Act was amended to enable the US Secretary of Agriculture to defend the country against any import which endangered national security, from Danish cheese to Turkish sultana raisins.[17]

Despite protection, the openness to direct investment by US transnational corporations helped to integrate European and US agro-food sectors via industrial inputs and processing. Both in promoting meat-intensive diets and in organizing intensive livestock production, agro-food capitals shaped agricultural reconstruction along lines similar to the US. Most important was investment in an intensive livestock sector relying on industrial feedstuffs composed from soy and maize. This linked apparently national agricultures to imported inputs. Beneath the protected surface, therefore, lay the corporate organization of a transnational agro-food complex centred on the Atlantic economy. It linked North America, especially the US, to Europe.[18]

The combination of the freedom of capital and the restriction of trade shaped agricultural reconstruction so that it created a new relationship between European and US agro-food sectors. A decade later, the Common Agricultural Policy of the European Community introduced a similar form of agricultural support to that in the US. To achieve import substitution in the face of chronic US surpluses, however, the level of protection required was very much higher. In return for the US acceptance of EEC restrictions against wheat and dairy imports (the old products in international trade), the EEC did not restrict the new US exports, maize and soy. The latter soon came to account for greater export revenues than those lost with wheat.[19] Both European corporations and subsidiaries of US corporations in Europe contributed to a massive growth of manufactured feedstuffs for intensive livestock production, and a shift from domestic and colonial raw materials, such as flax and cotton meal, to maize and soy imported from the US. Like other industrial sectors, the apparently national livestock industry rested on a chain of inputs which effectively integrated a transnational sector.[20]

Thus European wheat replicated the national US sector, while specialized European livestock farms imported inputs from the US, creating an integrated Atlantic agro-food sector. The price support mechanism for wheat and dairy products eventually replicated the surpluses, and with them the export subsidies to dispose of them. By 1975 the EC had switched from being a net importer to a net exporter of wheat, and by 1985, France's exports (including those to other EC members) were larger than those of the US.[21] At the same time, agro-industrial integration allowed European livestock producers to substitute a wide range of feed ingredients for US imports and to diversify trade. Eventually, the Common Agricultural Policy closed the circle by introducing support for domestic oilseed production, an import substitution/replication which eventually brought the US and EC to the brink of trade war in 1992.[22] Thus, trade restrictions and competitive dumping turned from the founding principle into the enduring friction of the food regime.

The Third World

The Atlantic agro-food economy was the hinge for the reconfiguration of the food relations of Asian, Latin American and African countries. As Third World states sought to develop national economies, their agrarian strategies were shaped by the opportunities and limits of world food markets. These gave little reason to question the dominant ideologies – capitalist and socialist; modernization and dependency – which all encouraged states to downplay agriculture except as a contribution to industrial development. For most countries, both the food supply of urban populations and the export revenues for industrial investment were largely sought outside traditional agrarian sectors during the 1950s and 1960s.

For the commercial food supply, US wheat surpluses made imports an attractive alternative to the modernization of the domestic food sector. When the US lost European wheat markets, which had been virtually the only source of import demand until the 1950s, it sought other outlets for its surpluses. It found them in Japan, and above all in the emerging Third World. Third World markets were cultivated, despite lack of foreign exchange, through the use of food aid. The main US food aid instrument, Public Law 480 (PL480), adapted the specific mechanisms invented for Marshall aid. However, while Marshall administrators in Europe had resisted the Congressional attempts to dump US wheat because it undermined the main goal of agricultural reconstruction,[23] there was no such counterbalance for PL480 aid in Third World countries. Consistent imports made many Third World countries dependent on cheap world wheat supplies.[24]

Wheat was both a change from most traditional dietary staples and an efficiently produced, often subsidized alternative to the marketed crops of domestic farmers. Despite the 'green revolution', which replicated in the Third World the hybrid maize revolution of US agriculture,[25] and integrated national agriculture into world markets for equipment and chemical inputs, the Third World as a whole became the main source of import demand on world wheat markets. Import policies created food dependence within two decades in countries which had been mostly self-sufficient in food at the end of World War II.

On the export side, tropical crops faced the notorious problem of declining terms of trade, even when export states tried to manage world supplies.[26] Two of the most important tropical export crops, sugar and vegetable oils, were increasingly marginalized by industrial substitutes used as sweeteners and oils. Although changing US (and other advanced country) diets increased the per capita consumption of sugars and fats, these were increasingly consumed in a new form. Sugars and fats became intermediate ingredients in manufactured foods rather than articles used directly by consumers.

Once industrial processes allowed for technical substitutions, the relative costs of crops could determine which would be used as raw materials for durable foods. The main industrial substitute for cane sugar was high fructose corn syrup, which became economically feasible to use because of US subsidies and surplus stocks of maize. The main substitute for tropical vegetable oils was soya oil, which was a byproduct of soymeal for animal feeds. Beyond that, soya oil was the second largest US food aid item after wheat, and was widely substituted for traditional oils for cooking and for industry, in recipients of US aid from Spain to India.[27] Thus the food regime fostered import substitution of tropical oils and sugars in the US and Europe, the Atlantic hinge of the international food regime.

By the early 1970s, then, the food regime had caught the Third World in a scissors. One blade was food import dependency. The other blade was declining revenues from traditional exports of tropical crops. If subsidized wheat surpluses were to disappear, maintaining domestic food supplies would depend on finding some other source of hard currency to finance imports.

The food crisis of 1973–4 did create a sudden scarcity. It sent prices soaring and dried up aid. Worst of all of dependent Third World importers, the food crisis coincided with the oil crisis.[28] The effects included a complex differentiation of the Third World based on the new importance of paying for expensive imports of food and energy. The solution was temporary, elegant and dangerous. The oil revenues deposited in transnational banks by oil-rich states were lent out extravagantly to states desperately in need of financing food (and oil) imports.

New Relations, New Rules, 1972–present

After two decades, the internal tensions within the food regime had begun to pose serious problems. The replication of surpluses, combined with the decline of the dollar as the international currency, led to competitive dumping and potential trade wars, particularly between the European Economic Community and the US. This eventually made it unbearably costly for small countries, such as Canada or Sweden, to subsidize surpluses or exports. On top of international conflict, transnational corporations outgrew the national regulatory frameworks in which they were born, and found them to be obstacles to further integration of a potentially global agro-food sector.

However, the crisis was precipitated externally by an event which permanently breached the boundary between the capitalist and socialist parts of the food regime. The geopolitical context for both Atlantic integration and the reorientation of Third World agro-food relations was Cold War rivalry. The catalyst of crisis in the early 1970s, a crisis from which the regime has yet to recover, was the massive grain deals between the US and the former USSR which accompanied detente. The crisis unfolded through a series of US embargoes in response to feared shortages throughout the 1970s, followed by fierce rivalry when chronic surpluses returned in the 1980s.

Detente and the Linking of Blocs

It will take a long time to interpret the effects of East–West relations on capitalism, but their role in the food regime was crucial. The food relations among the US, Europe, the Third World and, as we shall see, the Asian capitalist countries, were only one part, though the dominant part, of the food regime. They were contained by the Cold War dam which, despite leaks, divided the capitalist and the state socialist economies. With detente, major trade and financial links breached the Cold War dam. It is important to underscore that nearly two decades before the collapse of the socialist bloc and of the Soviet Union, economic ties between blocs had forever altered international food relations.

The Soviet–American grain deals of 1972 and 1973 permanently broke the dam separating capitalist and socialist blocs.[29] Despite leakages, this dam had been a wall containing the surpluses which were the pivot of the food regime. In the 1972–3 crop year, the Soviet Union bought 30 million metric tons of grain, which amounted to three-quarters of all commercially traded grain in the world.[30] The scale of that transaction created a sudden unprecedented shortage and skyrocketing prices. Even though surpluses returned in a few years because the agricultural commodity programmes which generated them remained in place, the tensions did not disappear, but were intensified by farm debt and state debt, international competition and the changing balance of power among states.

The sudden scarcity of grains and soybeans precipitated by the Soviet purchases provoked a counterproductive response by the US. First of all, despite 40 years of experience, the US Department of Agriculture acted as if the chronic surplus problem engendered by commodity price supports had disappeared. With state encouragement, US farmers abandoned conservation and other practices which had reduced acreage erratically since the New Deal. They followed the advice of the Secretary of Agriculture to plant 'fence-row to fence-row' to supply foreign demand for wheat, maize and soybeans. Although the US farm bill of 1973 finally introduced deficiency payments, target prices and other measures rejected in 1948 as an alternative to simple commodity price supports, the government also raised subsidies.[31] Hastily treating surpluses as a bad memory, farmers borrowed to finance expansion. In the US farm debt more than tripled in the 1970s, fuelled by high prices and speculation in farmland.[32]

Second, the Nixon administration, already beset by the Watergate scandals and nervous at the prospect of domestic feed shortages, introduced a series of embargoes between 1973 and 1975, which prevented internationally co-operative adjustments to the new conditions. The grain deal of 1972 was the economic centrepiece of its major foreign policy initiative, detente with the Soviet Union. This focus led to the shift of agricultural trade policy from the Department of Agriculture (as an adjunct to the farm programme) to the State Department, where it served US foreign policy as 'a lever that . . . has brought back into the world economy some 1.1 billion people' of the Soviet Union and People's Republic of China.[33] The US government gave the Soviets 75 per cent of allocated Concessionary

Commercial Credit (CCC) export credits, plus additional subsidies which reduced the export price below the domestic price. When the details became public, another scandal resulted in Congressional inquiries into the 'great Soviet grain robbery'.[34] When soybean prices began to climb the following year, consumers and livestock farmers mobilized, and the US embargoed all exports in July 1973. Then in 1974 and 1975, fearful of a repeat of the scandals of 1972, the US embargoed grain to the Soviet Union.[35]

The embargoes were complete failures. They revealed that the US government could not control trade even when, as for soybeans, the US had a virtual monopoly over supply. State trading agencies and transnational corporations and their subsidiaries were able to use complex transactions and trans-shipments to organize trade outside the knowledge, much less the control, of the US government or indeed of any state. Within two months of declaring the second embargo, the US negotiated the first of a series of five-year contracts with the Soviet Union.[36] This represented the largest single transaction in the world food economy.

This rapid US shift in 1975 implicitly acknowledged the frailty of US food surpluses as a weapon. The US reversed course by shifting the focus to economic policy intended to increase export earnings. By 1980 exports of grains and feeds had increased eight times over the 1970 level. The dependence of the US on agricultural exports was compounded by the fact that a quarter of its maize and about 15 per cent of its wheat was bought by the USSR.[37]

Nonetheless, the Carter administration imposed one last embargo in 1980 (despite its electoral pledge never to do so) in response to the Soviet invasion of Afghanistan. The Soviets bought almost the whole amount of the cancelled contracts on the world market, mostly from Argentina, Canada and possibly even the US via trans-shipments from Eastern Europe. Moreover, the Soviet Union had hard currency from its oil exports with which to buy grain and oilseeds. Consequently, the US embargo gave windfall prices to producers in competing export countries, and windfall profits to the corporate traders which took advantage of the unusual price fluctuations.[38] The disastrous embargo was one of the woes leading to the defeat of the Carter administration in the next election. Thus, even though the Soviet Union and Eastern Europe together accounted for imports valued at only a third of those of the Third World, the US became dependent on Soviet purchases.[39]

Yet within less than a decade the Soviet market, having risen to second largest in the world, effectively collapsed. Over the course of the 1980s, Soviet imports began to be sustained by the same US mercantile trade practices which had been applied earlier to Europe, Japan and the Third World. A high level of guarantees and bonuses, that is, subsidies, maintained Soviet purchases from the US in 1990 and 1991. As late as 12 December 1991, President Bush offered the USSR $1 billion dollars in credit guarantees for feedstuffs. Between 1987 and 1991, the US gave over $708 million in bonuses for Soviet wheat purchases. By then, subsidized sales by the US to the Soviet Union were such a large proportion of world trade that each transaction further depressed prices. Indeed, the US even revived a credit guarantee programme via the Export–Import Bank which had been defunct for 16 years in order to offer an additional $300 million in guarantees to the Soviet Union.[40] The former Soviet Union was on the list of 28 countries to receive subsidized exports announced by President Bush in September 1992 in his campaign for re-election in farm states. Short of getting the EC to agree to loss of major foreign and domestic markets, US policy now depends on increasing subsidized exports to cash-strapped countries whose prospects of repayment are dim.

Wheat, corn and soybean stocks in the US rose again in the 1980s, although new policies and expectations kept them in private hands.[41] When the surpluses returned, they were harder to dispose of than before the boom. The US had expanded its production and world market share instead of reforming agricultural policy.[42] US farmers carried a debt load which could not be supported when falling prices reduced cash flows and deflated land values, and in the 1980s farm failures became as severe as in the 1930s. Farmers had meanwhile lost many of their urban allies and their unity across commodity groups, making room for agro-food corporations to exercise the most effective lobby.[43] When the bubble burst in the 1980s, US farmers had lost their monopoly over agricultural exports, and their political weight in US trade policy.

Japan and the Asian Tigers

Just at the time when the US was becoming dependent on grain and soybean exports, its economic weight was declining relative to the EC and Japan, which were the major markets protected against its products. While the US and Europe were sliding into a subsidy war, relations between Japan and major exporters began to evolve in distinct ways. With the manifest collapse of the socialist bloc market after 1991, those relations revived the older, pre-war competition centred on import demand. These economic relations are deeply subversive of the defining principle of the food regime, namely power based on state-supported exports of surplus commodities.

Japan's national agro-food economy began with Marshall aid. The Allied Occupation carried out a land reform and created a large class of small farmers whose interests lay in maintaining high subsidies for rice. Japan's post-war agro-food reconstruction replicated the US model, adapted to the circumstances of rice production. Rice producers became politically important to successive governments, and the security afforded by domestic rice supplies became a tenet of national ideology. Subsequent US strategic aid to South Korea and Taiwan had similar effects.[44]

Yet replication was not balanced by integration as in Europe. Despite the similar goals and policies of Marshall aid, the economic and political conditions after the war, plus a lack of historical connections, led US corporations to shy away from significant direct investments in Japan of the sort they were undertaking in Europe.[45] Thus compared to Europe, US transnational firms did not create production chains integrating Japan's agro-food sector with that of the US.

In addition to post-war strategic conditions, the distinctively national character of the Japanese agro-food sector stemmed in part from its distinct diet. Although Japan early became a major importer of grains and soy, it played different roles in consumption and therefore in production. Wheat reflected a dietary change, encouraged by numerous trade missions and specific aid projects, such as provision of school meals. Japan became the largest of the new wheat importers after World War II, the rest being countries of the emerging Third World. By incorporating wheat into their diets, Japanese consumers benefited from low world prices and helped clear US surpluses from the market. In this sense, Japan played the same role as Third World countries in restructuring international wheat trade around the US as an export centre.

Japan's relation to international soy markets was also different from that of Europe. Since soy was initially used mainly for human diets, it did not enter the economic and technical chains of the feedstuffs industry. The manufacture of soybeans into tofu, miso and other foods was a distinct, Japanese production. Most important, as human food, soy cannot be substituted in the way that animal feeds can be – and eventually were. By the time Japan began to import significant quantities of soy for animal feeds, the food regime was already changing.

Dependence on US imports was reliable during the stable period of the food regime, when US surpluses led to cheap world supplies. However, the US soy embargo of 1973 changed Japanese perceptions radically and permanently. Although the embargo lasted only two months and all contracts were eventually honoured, its effect on the confidence of import states was enduring.[46] In particular, the embargo fatefully impressed the government of Japan with the unreliability of the US as a source of virtually all its soy. By 1980, as we shall see, the US share of world soya markets plummeted from its virtual monopoly a decade earlier. US trade negotiations with Japan in the subsequent two decades have included repeated but fruitless apologies for that political blunder more than twenty years ago.[47] This may be the reason that US pressure on Japan to reduce agricultural trade barriers in the early 1980s concentrated on beef and citrus products, rather than rice.[48]

Japan's investment and trade became a major force in the transformation.

Japanese agro-food investments abroad began after the food crisis. If we understand soy and grains to be resources necessary for the domestic economy, then they may fall under the larger resource strategy described for minerals by Bunker and O'Hearn. According to their account, Japan and the US have consistently adopted completely different foreign economic strategies, based on their distinct endowments of natural resources.[49] They argue that without significant domestic production, the Japanese interest is in diversity of supply, which keeps prices down and reduces strategic dependence on any supplier. Japan can best achieve this goal by using the minimum investment necessary to create as many export sectors as possible. Exporters then compete for the Japanese import market, and Japanese importers can pick and choose, and shift from one supplier to another. This contrasts sharply with the longstanding US (and European) pattern of direct foreign investment. Both domestic production by US corporations, and foreign production by their subsidiaries, are locked into production sites and technologies matched to those sites.[50]

Unlike the US, and even the European Community, Japan is destined to import soy. The component of soy imports used in human diets is not substitutable. With the crucial exception of rice, imports of many agricultural products, and especially soy, are as important to Japan as minerals. In addition to the central tenet of agricultural policy, which continues to be national sufficiency in rice, Japan's interest as an importer lies unambiguously in secure access to necessary imports of grains and soy.

Although Japan is a distant second to the European Community in the volume of its soy and feedgrain imports, its singular foreign economic strategy has the potential completely to undermine the structure of international food relations. Japan began in the early 1970s to look for alternative sources of soy supply to the US. Its strategy was to change the nature of surpluses from a problem of disposal, which the US and EC confronted, to an advantage for the buyer. It found a complementary interest among countries of the Third World whose national industrial policies created internationally competitive agro-food sectors in the 1960s and after.

New Agricultural Countries

Behind the scenes of the Atlantic conflict which held centre stage at the GATT, there is a new alignment. Trade between Japan (and other commercial importers) and successful new agro-food exporters in the Third World continues to destabilize the Atlantic-centred food regime. The new relations began during the early crisis years of the 1970s.

Soviet–American trade brought skyrocketing prices and new export markets in the 1970s. These conditions coincided with the new possibilities for public borrowing created by the oil crisis.[51] OPEC (Organization of Petroleum Exporting Countries) states captured a large share of world revenues and deposited them in international banks. The banks in turn pressed these 'petrodollars' on borrowers. Many of the borrowers were Third World and socialist states, including some which hoped to invest in export agriculture and to use the earnings to repay the loans. Another set of borrowers, on a scale equivalent to Third World debt, was US farmers. Lending of petrodollars in the 1970s fuelled both buyers and sellers of an expanding world market.

The differentiation of the Third World into oil exporters, successful exporters of manufactured products and those left behind in poverty (sometimes called the 'Fourth World'), began in the early 1970s. The new industrial countries, called NICs, were part of a transnational restructuring of industrial production. As we have seen, the technical basis of the American model of agriculture, which was replicated and integrated in different ways in other parts of the world, comprised the subordination of crops and livestock into corporate, often transnational, agro-food complexes and the industrialization of agriculture itself. The successful development of export agriculture was as important as that of manufactures, and created a comparable set of 'new agricultural countries', or NACs. Some, such as Brazil, are both NICs and NACs.

Brazil is the most important NAC. Its export capacity was based on a particularly successful development of the industrial agro-food economy in the 1960s, by means of state-guided policies of industrialization through import substitution. Starting in the 1960s, the Brazilian state used a strategic mix of agricultural settlement, credit and taxation policies to create an intensive livestock sector based on nationally produced grain and soya. Not only that, but export taxes on unprocessed soya encouraged national processing, whether by state or private, national or translational corporations.

Brazil replicated and modernized the US model of state-organized agro-food production. It shifted the focus of domestic policy from agricultural subsidies to agro-industry, which increased the value of commodities and did not create surpluses. Brazilian export policy replaced the US focus on the stabilization of domestic farm programmes, with an emphasis on high value-added exports.[52]

Within four years of the US soy embargo of 1973, NACs had cut into the previous virtual US export monopoly. By 1977, the US share of world exports of oilseeds and meals, of which soy was the largest, was only 54.6 per cent.[53] Ten years later, the US share of world oilmeal exports had fallen to one-sixth. It exported less than Brazil and only slightly more than Argentina. China, Chile and India had joined the ranks of major oilmeal exporters.[54]

Ironically, the US retained a nearly two-thirds share of unprocessed oilseed exports, while Brazil exported high value-added meal. When Japan, the Soviet Union and other import countries looked for alternatives to US supplies, Brazil was especially well poised to concentrate on value-added meal rather than unprocessed soybeans. By 1980 Brazilian soybean production was a third as large as that of the US, and its soymeal production half as large; Brazilian exports of soybeans were 10 per cent of US exports, but its soymeal exports were virtually equal. Then within a few years, as mentioned above, Brazilian soymeal exports exceeded those of the US.[55]

Thus, Brazil's successful adaptation of the US model, which shifted the focus from agriculture to agro-industry and from the management of surpluses to commercial exports, involved a complex web of international and social transformations. It gave Brazil a competitive advantage in a technically evolving and increasingly open international food economy – at a high cost to the victims of capitalist transformation of the agro-food economy of Brazil.[56] Most important for international food relations, the NAC phenomenon revives the intense export competition on world markets that existed prior to the post-war food regime, and shifts advantage from exporters to importers.

This fitted neatly with Japanese strategies to diversify world supplies with minimal investments and commitments abroad. Like many other states caught in the debt trap, as Bunker and O'Hearn point out, public investments and joint ventures in Third World export sectors allowed Japanese capital to gain leverage with minimal direct investment. This link between Third World states and (often Japanese) foreign capital supplanted the earlier combination of direct (US and European) foreign investment and state investment and controls favouring import substitution.

Liberalization has created an unstable situation in which importers (with strong currencies) benefit and the largest exporter wields the greatest power in international rule-making. Paradoxically, liberal trade practices now so desperately pursued by the US to manage short-term deficits, reinforce the long-term shift of advantage to (economically strong) importing countries. With success at the GATT the US could find itself in a new set of international relations, in which the rules convert export surpluses from a source of power into a source of dependency.

The End of the Surplus Regime

The impasse over agricultural subsidies at the Uruguay Round of GATT reflected the contradictory foundations of the post-war food regime, foundations which are crumbling rapidly. Overt conflict between the replication and integration of national agro-food sectors at the end of 1992 was reduced to a few million tons of oilseeds. That it was important enough to jeopardize the comprehensive multilateral agreement to extend corporate power in key sectors for future accumulation, such as services and intellectual property rights, testifies to the strength of residual tendencies in the food regime. Even the 1993 agreements to reduce European Community subsidies and end mercantile trade rules, do not assure the future envisioned in the larger GATT agreements. The contest will continue between political projects involving different future scenarios.

The End of Commodity Programmes?

Farm policies were catching up with the collapse of the post-war food regime even before the GATT agreement. Changes in agricultural policy unimaginable at the outset of the Uruguay Round anticipate an end to national surpluses.

The separation of farm income supports from production – that is, the end of price supports – is the likely future for North America and Europe. This would undo the key feature replicated in the food regime – government-generated surpluses. In the US, although farm lobbies gained provisions requiring the reinstatement of old measures if the Uruguay Round breaks down, the farm bill of 1985 accelerated the shift from price to income supports – even as it intensified export subsidies.[57] After 1987, fiscal pressures reduced the level of price supports. Most of the states which are the stronghold of the farm lobby voted Republican in the November 1992 US elections, and the Democratic incumbent may feel less beholden to them than the past decade's ruling Republicans. In the European Community, reforms of the Common Agricultural Policy initiated in 1988 and intensified in 1991, point more decisively in the same direction. Payments to farmers will support their incomes directly, instead of indirectly through the prices of their commodities. While farmers will no doubt continue to be forced off the land, at least some will be supported as a combined rural welfare and tourism project. Farm income supports may also be tied to the management of rural resources and to environmental programmes.[58]

The shift to income supports promises eventually to end the mountains and lakes of surplus agricultural commodities disposed of abroad by means of government subsidies and credits. It is easy to ignore the remarkable consensus over this way of ending an epoch of agricultural policy because (at least to proponents of urgent liberalization) implementation seems glacial.[59] Yet the shift is likely to continue, because it confirms in policy what has already occurred structurally. Whatever stocks may be intentionally created for stabilization or security, whatever export subsidies and import controls may be retained or introduced, will have – indeed already do have – effects on the global agro-food sector different from those which shaped the food regime.

The Food Regime Unhinged

The two trade hinges of the food regime are coming loose. Countries of the Third World and, more recently, of the former socialist bloc, have joined the multilateral trade negotiations at the GATT.[60] This reflects (and reinforces) the unhinging of Atlantic agro-food integration, and of the US–Third World grain trade.

The Atlantic hinge is weakening as Western Europe and the US are reorienting trade towards their respective continents. The North American Free Trade Agreement (NAFTA) of 1992 and the potential expansion of the European Community to Nordic, former socialist and other countries, promises to extend 'decoupling' to the continents of North America and Europe. This has been envisioned by corporate policy advocates for some time. As early as 1987, the President of Cargill Ltd. told the leading Canadian financial journal: 'Major agricultural producing countries should concentrate on devising actuarially sound income insurance policies . . . but we must avoid like the plague commodity-specific programs that encourage overproduction or distort land use decisions.'[61] Continental integration is also emerging in Asia, centred on Japanese imports and investment.[62] Whether these turn out to be rivals or partners, they replace the US centre of the food regime with multiple centres.

The Atlantic hinge held because of the Cold War division of Europe. The collapse of the socialist bloc was crucial in breaking the impasse over West European farm policy, by separating reform of the Common Agricultural Policy from the conflict with the US. The prospective incorporation into the European Community of Eastern Europe (and new Nordic and Alpine members), according to Tim Josling, was the most compelling reason for the MacSharry reform proposals.[63] The former socialist countries include large fertile regions, which are politically divided, economically underdeveloped and culturally distinct. Much like the American South in the 1950s and 1960s, where soy rapidly replaced cotton, it opens a rich hinterland with abundant land and labour for reconstructing continental agro-food relations. If stability returns to the former Soviet Union, the indiscriminately maligned state and collective farms may provide ripe pickings for agro-food transnationals (not only European-based, of course), particularly in the livestock sector. Similar openings could include China in a Japanese diversification of investment and trade.

The other hinge was between the US on one side, and the Third World (and Japan) on the other. The decline of US economic power parallels the transformation of exports from a source of power into a source of dependence. US exports were a source of economic and strategic power. In many underdeveloped countries, the food regime left a legacy of food import dependence, stagnating export revenues and debt. Later, a few became

NACs, whose competitive exports helped to disrupt the food regime. Now, in the twilight of the regime, the export imperative prevails. For strong importing economies, such as Japan, this is an advantage. For the Third World as a whole, the transformation of their economies into agricultural export platforms intensifies new global international hierarchies between North and South.[64]

The export imperative completely undermines US centrality in the food regime. The 'inevitable trend toward export dependence'[65] which was built into US farm and export-and-aid programmes, has come to its fruition. For a decade, Republican governments in the US have sacrificed long-term restructuring to aggressive export practices. The US zeal to force open commercial markets implicitly recognized the failure of concessional sales, long-term credits and other forms of 'aid' to create new markets. Surpluses have come to signify weakness rather than power, a burden rather than an opportunity.[66] The need for markets and the need to restructure domestic agriculture have led to contradictory foreign economic policy – aggressive trade practices combined (since 1987) with insistent demands to abolish such practices.

The accession of former Third World countries into the GATT and their sudden conversion to free trade signals the subordination of food restructuring to relations of international debt.[67] The promotion of agricultural exports, especially those called 'non-traditional' (geared to new niche markets for exotic foods, flowers and other crops), is an explicit aim of structural adjustment conditions imposed by creditors. They usually intensify social inequalities and conflicts in poor countries. For instance, Brazil, which is a stunning success as measured by investment in agro-food production and exports, is also a nightmare of evictions from the land, displacement of local food systems, hunger and social unrest.[68] At the time of writing, major social unrest has precipitated massive food distribution to the poor. This food intervention is certainly less orderly and less integrated with public policy than were the food subsidies abolished in the past decade of austerity.[69] These popular reactions are part of a string of 'IMF riots', frequently over food prices, during the past decade of austerity.[70] They reflect the suffering imposed in new centres of accumulation like Brazil, no less than in the vast regions pushed to the margins of accumulation, which include much of the African continent.

Debtor countries are caught in a scissors between the export imperative and import restrictions in Northern markets. They are thus forced to support free trade, however difficult is the shift from decades of import substitution, controlled flows of goods and money, and state enterprises. Debt repayment and currency reform require access to highly protected food markets in North America, Europe and Japan. Liberal capitalism is the new, externally imposed form of austerity in the late twentieth century. It is in marked contrast to the austerity chosen by revolutionary Third World states of the Cold War era, which took the form of autarkic socialism. Collectivization regardless of national circumstances was often futile and even disastrous. The same can be said of the creation of agro-food export platforms regardless of national circumstances.

Two tendencies have emerged since the Uruguay Round began in 1986, which prefigure alternative rules and politics of food. One is the project of corporate freedom contained in the new GATT rules. The other is less formed: a set of projects developing from the politics of environment, diet, livelihood and democratic control over economic life. Farmers must somehow ally themselves in the main contest over future regulation: will it be mainly private and corporate, or public and democratic? What international rules would promote each alternative? The answers depend on the ways that emerging agro-food policies are linked either to capital accumulation or to demands raised by popular social movements.

Private Global Regulation?

At present, agro-food corporations are the major agents attempting to regulate agro-food conditions, that is, to organize stable conditions of production and consumption which allow them to plan investment, sourcing of agricultural raw materials and marketing.[71] The new rules defined by the December 1993 GATT agreement significantly empower transnational capital. This empowerment concerns not only the freedom to trade and invest in agriculture (cattle and potatoes), industry (frozen hamburgers and chips) and services (hot hamburgers and chips). Provisions for intellectual property rights also have serious implications for uses of biotechnologies, for control over genetic resources and for standards protecting craft and regional foods.[72]

However, transnational agro-food corporations have now outgrown the regime that spawned them. In particular, even US-based corporations have long had interests of their own, not related to those of the US state or national economy, and certainly not to those of US farmers.[73] A major reason why US embargoes never worked, for instance, was corporate collusion with importing countries to evade US trade restrictions.[74] Even before the food crisis, subsidiaries of US corporations were working independently of US national policy. For instance, in 1970, subsidiaries of Cargill and Continental, assisted by a trade agency of the French government, joined with other major grain companies in a cartel, Francéréales, to promote French exports. The cartel was dissolved in 1973, under pressure from public authorities and from excluded competitors, but was revived in 1975 to respond to the new Soviet market.[75] Because the US state could not control or even monitor shipments by transnational corporations, US policies to increase US food exports at the same time undercut US political power.

Within the limits of international rules, the corporate integration of a global agro-food sector has proceeded as quickly and thoroughly as changing technologies permit. A new degree of global sourcing is made possible by feedstuffs that substitute for the standard corn and soy combination of the food regime.[76] Two examples may suggest how 'substitute feeds' at once integrate agro-food complexes and render substitutable the exports (and farmers) of any nation. First, orange pulp, a byproduct of the frozen orange juice industry, integrates the livestock and durable foods complexes. This adds complexity to the competition between Brazil and the US, which includes (among others) an interplay between now-traditional feeds (soy) and durable foods (frozen juice). Second, complex commercial relations surround corn gluten as a substitute feed. This product, which is highly protected by the European Community, is the byproduct of the manufacture of high fructose corn syrup. The latter is the main sugar substitute in food manufacture. Without export revenues from gluten feed, the use of corn as a sweetener is too costly, and the domestic US demand for corn will fall considerably. Not surprisingly, this was one of the European import duties most intensely contested by the US.[77]

Meanwhile, as the rules are shifting, so are the commodities central to capital accumulation. While feedstuffs, the heart of the food regime, are becoming globalized rather than merely internationalized, the completely new markets in 'exotic' fruits and vegetables are global from the outset. Any state can enter, and in the push and shove of new markets, there is room for fly-by-night entrepreneurs and instant transnational corporations, as well as the giants of the post-war agro-food regime.[78] Rapacious entrepreneurial practices are encouraged by slavish state policies to attract investments and promote exports. The paradise of eternal strawberries and ornamental plants for rich consumers depends on an underworld of social disruption and ecological irresponsibility. Whilst no rules have yet stabilized 'non-traditional' export markets, the main corporate agenda points to global sourcing and marketing, that is, the impulse to diversify suppliers and cultivate tastes for 'exotic' foods (pears in Mexico no less than starfruit in Canada). Superimposed on the diversification of raw materials for mass-produced durable foods is this post-Fordist scenario of 'flexible specialization' and 'niche markets'.

Democratic Public Regulation?

Stable rules cannot come from private and competitive organizations, despite the global reach of some corporations. There are two reasons for this. First, the very conditions which allowed for agro-food capitals to become pivots of accumulation have created new social actors and new social problems. Second, agro-food corporations are actually heterogeneous in their interests.

Classes of producers and consumers have changed radically from the time when transnational agro-food corporations were born. The agro-food sector is now focused on food – industry and services – rather than on agriculture. The character of classes, urban and rural, involved in food production has shifted. In meat-packing, for instance, the scale of production has increased dramatically. This has been accompanied by massive restructuring of the labour process and a standardization of products. The main result in the US over the past two decades has been to replace a native-born, male workforce – both assembly line workers in packing plants and skilled butchers in supermarkets – with new immigrants, often female, recruited to work in new plants in small cities in the US plains.[79] Restructuring is occurring as well in Australia, mainly for export to the Pacific Rim, at massive environmental cost.[80] Both cases echo in the old centres of accumulation a process that began in NACs, such as Mexico, of creating the 'world steer' at the expense of the traditional markets for peasant sideline production of cattle.[81]

As farmers have declined in numbers and unity, and workers have lost some of their bargaining power with agro-food corporations, food politics have shifted to urban issues, that is, to *food* rather than *agriculture*. Consumers in the food regime have been educated by agro-food corporations to desire first standard foods, and then exotic foods from the entire globe. Yet more contradictions have emerged in the sphere of consumption. Poverty limits access to food and demand for the products of the agro-food economy. In the poorest parts of the world, and the poorest populations of rich countries, many are forced to withdraw from commodity relations into self-provisioning and informal networks of exchange. More privileged consumers have come to appreciate the dangers to health and environment from the dominant practices of agro-food production created by the food regime – mainly the chemical-intensive monocultures of farming and the chemical-intensive production of durable foods. The most privileged consumers have revived demand for handcrafted goods, including meals, now expressed in the language of 'designer' foods.

A food policy is more adequate for the present circumstances than the farm policies left behind by the waning food regime. It is made possible by the decoupling of farm incomes from agricultural production. The national agricultural policies of the food regime not only supported prices and generated surpluses. Through credit and insurance criteria, for instance, they also fostered large farms, monocultural practices and the environmentally destructive use of chemicals and heavy machinery. They also encouraged the technological and social dependence of farmers on corporate suppliers of packages of chemical inputs and purchasers of contractually specified crops and animals. As national farm policies come under increasing pressure, the possibility arises to create a democratic food policy.

The social basis for a democratic food policy lies in movements for employment and incomes, for safe and nutritious food, for environmentally sustainable agriculture (including humane treatment of animals) and for democratic participation. The main social movements concerned with aspects of food focus on poverty, hunger, employment, health, cultural integrity, the environment, rural recreation and even animal rights. Within this field of issues, agricultural regulation could become part of a comprehensive plan to use the capacities of people and the land to meet social needs for nourishment, cultural expression and a congenial habitat.

A democratic food policy is quite a different prospect from the implicit policy posited by liberalization of trade and empowerment of transnational corporations. The latter moves beyond the global promotion of American diets, such as hamburgers and cola drinks, to the creation of a global diet consisting of an array of manufactured meals and ingredients, called Chinese, Mexican, Middle Eastern or whatever, in the freezers of supermarkets throughout the world. In so doing, it embodies principles of distance and durability.

Democratic principles, by contrast, emphasize proximity and seasonality. This means the use and development of technologies and markets to facilitate local enterprises in every possible link of agro-food chains. What is increasingly politically proposed is that healthy food and environmentally sound agriculture must be rooted in local economies. These must respond to the capacities and limits of agro-ecological regions, including the needs and capacities of the people who dwell there. In other words, food to nourish people and communities can only be linked to sustainable agriculture by means of chains of commerce and processing located as much as possible within regions. A democratic food policy can reconstruct the social, cultural and ecological diversity destroyed by the monocultural regions and transnational integration of the food regime.

At the same time, the heterogeneity of corporate interests suggests potential allies to support such policies at the national level. National states can protect and link regional projects if pressed to do so. Indeed, some of the most progressive technical possibilities, such as the substitution of fossil fuels by ethanol, depend entirely on the present structure of subsidies and protection. Even if that specific structure cannot be saved, important fractions of capital are engaged in long-term projects, such as Archer-Daniel Midlands in the US and Ferruzzi in Europe, whose interests, at least in part, lie in public regulation of agro-food economies.[82]

This possibility could only be pursued through institutions at all levels, from the municipal to the international. In various parts of the world, municipal and regional governments – or popular organizations – are experimenting with ways to support regional agro-food networks. These include community kitchens, support for scientific research geared to local food industries, and publicly supported community catering in schools and other public institutions.[83] With the exception of Sweden, however, no national state has undertaken to create a food policy as a framework for reshaping agriculture to meet environmental and social needs.[84] On the contrary, perhaps the most comprehensive national food system in the capitalist world is in an advanced stage of dismemberment in Mexico. A public corporation, whose activities extended beyond the regulation of agricultural prices into processing, distribution and the provision of affordable food to low-income consumers, effectively 'decoupled' from the market rights to land and rights to food.[85] Against popular resistance, whose scale and intensity are not yet evident, a decade ago new political elites began to dismantle the Mexican system under pressure of negotiated austerity measures and anticipated continental free trade.

Even with national support, the success of regional agro-food systems depends on international institutions. The World Food Board proposal of 1947, which expressed the hopes of a war-torn and hungry world for international co-operation to plan food and agriculture, belongs to the past.[86] But it is important to remember that alternatives did exist and choices were made. Despite the multiplication of the number of states since 1947, when many were part of European colonial empires or of the emerging Soviet bloc, virtually all countries participate in multilateral economic negotiations. Most are doing so at the very time when national states are being restructured in response to transnational capital.[87] The outcome depends on whether, despite their variety and inequality, movements for livelihood and democracy can shape the contest over new international rules, both within and outside the proposed World Trade Organization.

NOTES

1 Josling, Tim (1992) 'Emerging agricultural trade relations in the post Uruguay Round world', Paper presented at the Faculty of Political Science, University of Rome, June.

2 Nothing could be farther from the case. For instance, the whole edifice of the food regime would never have been constructed if the Brannan Plan – defeated in 1947 through intense redbaiting – had become the basis of US agricultural policy. See Christenson, Reo M. (1959) *The Brannan Plan: farm politics and policy*, Ann Arbor, University of Michigan Press.

3 The proposal for a World Food Board was defeated at a meeting in Washington, DC in August 1947. See Peterson, Martin (1990) 'Paradigmatic shift in agriculture: global effects and the Swedish response', in Terry Marsden, Philip Lowe and Sarah Whatmore (eds) *Rural Restructuring*, London, David Fulton, pp. 77–100.

4 For an exception, see Strange, Marty (1988) *Family Farming, A New Economic Vision*, Omaha, University of Nebraska Press, pp. 17–30.

5 While the US had been a major exporter in the earlier food regime of 1870–1939, it had shared dominance with Russia before the Revolution of 1917, and

then with faster growing exports from elsewhere, particularly the British Empire. The collapse of US exports in the Great Depression was more severe than other exporters. Consequently, its post-war dominance was by no means a continuation of a stable historical pattern. See Friedmann, H. (1978) 'World market, state, and family farm: social bases of household production in the era of wage labor', *Comparative Studies in Society and History* 20, 4.

6 Rau, Allen (1957) *Agricultural Policy and Trade Liberalization in the United States, 1934–56: a study of conflicting policies*, Geneva, Librairie E. Droz, pp. 93–121.

7 Ibid.

8 See Kenney, Martin, Lobao, Linda, M., Curry, James and Goe, W. Richard (1991) 'Agriculture in U.S. Fordism: the integration of the productive consumer', in William H. Friedland, Lawrence Busch, Frederick H. Buttel and Alan P. Rudy (eds) *Towards a New Political Economy of Agriculture*, Boulder, CO, Westview Press, pp. 173–88. In the same volume, see Berlan, Jean-Pierre, 'The historical roots of the present agricultural crisis', pp. 115–36, for analysis of the arable–livestock divide; and Buttel, Frederick H. and La Ramée, Pierre, 'The "disappearing middle": a sociological perspective', for differentiation of US farms by size.

9 The use of these foods was bound up with the new social relations of consumption based on purchases of appliances, such as refrigerators and freezers, by both stores and households. Hayden, Dolores (1984) *Redesigning the American Dream*, New York, Norton.

10 Bertrand, Jean-Pierre, Laurent, Catherine and LeClercq, Vincent (1983) *Le monde du soja*, Paris, Editions La Découverte.

11 See Gertler, Michael Eden (1991) 'The institutionalization of grower–processor relations in the vegetable industries of Ontario and New York', in Friedland et al. (eds) *Towards a New Political Economy*, pp. 232–55. See also Friedland, William H., Barton, Amy E. and Thomas, Robert J. (1981) *Manufacturing Green Gold: capital, labor, and technology in the lettuce industry*, Cambridge, Cambridge University Press.

12 Goodman, David, Sorj, Bernardo and Wilkinson, John (1987) *From Farming to Biotechnology*, Oxford, Blackwell Publishers.

13 For instance, Revel, Alain and Riboud, Christophe (1986) *America's Green Power*, Baltimore, Johns Hopkins University Press; Tubiana, Laurence (1989) 'World trade in agricultural products: from global regulation to market fragmentation', in David Goodman and Michael Redclift (eds) *International Farm Crisis*, London, Macmillan, pp. 23–45; George, Susan (1981) *Les stratèges de la faim*, Geneva, Editions Grounauer, especially pp. 23–56; Moore Lappe, Frances and Collins, Joseph (1986) *World Hunger, Twelve Myths*, San Francisco, Food First, p. 107.

14 Bertrand et al., *Le monde du soja*; Gilmore, Richard (1982) *A Poor Harvest: the clash of policies and interests in the grain trade*, New York and London, Longman.

15 Rau, *Agricultural Policy*.

16 Friedmann, H. (1990) 'Origins of Third World food dependence', in Henry Bernstein, Ben Crow, Maureen Mackintosh and Charlotte Martin (eds) *The Food Question*, London, Earthscan.

17 Rau, *Agricultural Policy*.

18 Bertrand et al., *Le monde du soja*.

19 Morgan, Dan (1979) *Merchants of Grain*, New York, Viking.
20 Morgan, *Merchants of Grain* and Bertrand et al., *Le monde du soja*.
21 Hathaway, Dale E. (1977) *Agriculture and the GATT: rewriting the rules*, Washington, DC, Institute for International Economics, p. 45.
22 It would be useful to investigate the role of European-based transnationals, such as Ferruzzi, in this policy change. It is interesting to recall that soybeans were included in US farm programmes at the behest of corporations wanting a stable supply of oil for margarine production.
23 Rau, *Agricultural Policy*, pp. 93–121.
24 Friedmann, 'Origins'.
25 Kloppenberg, Jr, Jack (1984) 'The social impacts of biogenetic technology in agriculture: past and future', in G. Berardi and C. Geisler (eds) *The Social Consequences and Challenges of New Agricultural Technologies*, Boulder, CO, Westview Press, pp. 291–321.
26 Friedmann, 'Origins' and Friedmann, H. (1991) 'Changes in the international division of labor', in Friedland et al. (eds) *Towards a New Political Economy*.
27 Friedmann, 'Changes in the international division of labor'.
28 The oil and food crises were connected. While the Soviet intention to import feedgrains resulted from an internal political decision to increase domestic meat consumption, their ability to do so was based on the hard currency earnings from their oil exports. The volume of revenues was very much due to the oil price rises set by the OPEC cartel. See Friedmann, H. (forthcoming) 'Warsaw Pact Socialism: detente and economic tensions in the Soviet bloc', in Allen Hunter (ed.) *Rethinking the Cold War*, Pittsburgh, Temple University Press.
29 Most accounts of the 'food crisis' list the Soviet purchases along with a variety of other factors, which coincided in the early 1970s to change the relation between supply and demand. These included, for instance, the failure of the Peruvian anchovy harvest, an important protein supplement in animal feeds. However, in a regime governed by chronic oversupply and rapid technical change, the opening of world demand to include the socialist bloc was clearly more significant for the structural basis of the regime.
30 Gilmore, *A Poor Harvest*, p. 227.
31 Gilmore, *A Poor Harvest*, pp. 75–7. For the historical alternative, see Christenson, *The Brannan Plan*.
32 Strange, *Family Farming*, pp. 21–2
33 Earl Butz, quoted in Gilmore, *A Poor Harvest*, p. 157.
34 Gilmore, *A Poor Harvest*, p. 75.
35 Ibid., pp. 146–60.
36 Ibid., pp. 159–60.
37 Revel and Riboud, *America's Green Power*, p. 173.
38 Gilmore, *A Poor Harvest*, pp. 165–9.
39 Organization for Economic Co-operation and Development (1991) *Agricultural Policies, Markets and Trade, Monitoring and Outlook*, Paris, OECD, p. 402.
40 United States Department of Agriculture, Economic Research Service (1991) *USSR Agriculture and Trade Report*, RS-91-1, May, p. 30.
41 See Strange, *Family Farming*, p. 23.
42 Revel and Riboud, *America's Green Power*, *passim*.
43 Gilmore, *A Poor Harvest*, p. 5.

44 McMichael, Philip and Kim, Chul-Kyoo (forthcoming) 'The restructuring of the agricultural systems of Japan and South Korea in comparative and global perspective', in Philip McMichael (ed.) *The Global Restructuring of Agro-food Systems*, Ithaca, NY, Cornell University Press.

45 Schonberger, H. B. (1989) *Aftermath of War: Americans and the remaking of Japan, 1945–1952*, Kent, OH, Kent State University Press.

46 Revel and Riboud, *America's Green Power*, p. 145.

47 Stephen Bunker, University of Wisconsin, personal communication.

48 Reich, Michael and Endo, Yasuo (1983) 'Conflicting demands in US–Japan agricultural negotiations', USJP Working Paper 83–01, Harvard University Center for International Affairs, May.

49 Bunker, Stephen and O'Hearn, Denis (1992) 'Strategies of economic ascendants for access to raw materials: a comparison of the U.S. and Japan', in Ravi Arvind Palat (ed.) *Pacific Asia and the Future of the World System*, Westport Greenwood Press. Bunker and O'Hearn show how, in the minerals sector, US transnational investment strategy eventually became a competitive disadvantage relative to the Japanese strategy of indirect control through minimal investment in multiple sources of supply. While US transnationals were tied to specific places and technologies, Japanese trade and investment could be used to induce Third World states to invest public money in infrastructure and even direct production for export of aluminium and other minerals. Third World nationalist responses to US hegemony fitted nicely with this strategy. By the time it became clear that the aggregate effects of national mineral projects were counterproductive, many Third World states were caught in the debt trap. Export-oriented industrialization reinforced their commitment to projects undertaken to industrialize through import substitution. As technologies and profitable sites changed, Japan could shift sources of supply, while vertically integrated US firms were stuck with devalued land and capital.

50 Ibid.

51 Friedmann, 'Warsaw Pact socialism'.

52 LeClercq, Vincent (1988) *Conditions et limites de l'insertion du Brésil dans les échanges mondiaux du soja*, Institut National de Recherches Agronomiques, Etudes et Recherches No. 96, Montpellier, Ecole Nationale Supérieure Agronomique.

53 Revel and Riboud, *America's Green Power*, p. 193.

54 Hathaway, *Agriculture and the GATT*, table 3.14, p. 52.

55 Ibid., p. 52; Bertrand et al., *Le monde du soja*, p. 16.

56 LeClercq, Vincent (1989) 'Aims and constraints of the Brazilian agro-industrial strategy: the case of Brazil', in Goodman and Redclift (eds) *International Farm Crisis*, pp. 275–91.

57 An intriguing argument has been made that the aggressive US stand was initiated by the US farm lobby in a strategy to *keep US farm programmes*. According to this view, the lobby was initiated and pressed for the 1987 US 'zero-option' demand for total abolition of all subsidies within ten years. The goal was to legislate reinstatement in case of failure, and to provoke the EC into rejection, thus ensuring failure. The game may work, but it may also backfire, the argument continues. If agreement is secured – not the zero-option but something wildly beyond what was thought to be possible in 1987 – then the US farm lobby is caught in a legislative and ideological trap of its own

making. See Paarlbert, Robert L. 'Why agriculture blocked the Uruguay Round: evolving strategies in a two level game', MS, Harvard Center for International Affairs, 26 March 1991.

58 Ironically, deficiency payments were the cornerstone of British agricultural policy before entry into the Common Agricultural Policy. Whilst they may be considered a welfare measure, subsidized via taxes and not affecting imports or prices, the recipients were members of the only national class of capitalist farmers in the world. The subsequent experience of the CAP, which enriched farmers and rewarded scale, makes it difficult to remember this rational policy.

59 OECD, *Agricultural Policies*, pp. 199–200.

60 See Josling, 'Emerging agricultural trade' and Josling (1992) 'Conflicts between free trade and domestic policies in agriculture and the environment', Paper presented at the Faculty of Political Science, University of Rome, May. Josling's account of the relationship between international changes and the GATT negotiations is remarkably insightful and pragmatic, and informs my account. However, despite his recognition that ' "new" trade is based not on old-style comparative advantage, based on resource endowment, but on intra-industry specialization, intra-firm investment decisions, and niche markets' ('Emerging agricultural trade', p. 4), Josling does not really incorporate economic power into his analysis.

61 *Financial Post*, 26 January 1987, quoted in Kneen, Brewster (1990) *Trading Up: how Cargill, the world's largest grain company, is changing Canadian agriculture*, Toronto, NC Press, p. 112.

62 McMichael, Philip (1992) 'Agro-food restructuring in the Pacific Rim', in Palat (ed.) *Pacific Asia*. Also Lawrence, Geoffrey and Vanclay, Frank (forthcoming) 'Agricultural change and environmental degradation in the semi-periphery: the Murray-Darling Basin, Australia', in P. McMichael (ed.) *Agro-food System Restructuring in the Late Twentieth Century*, Ithaca, NY, Cornell University Press. Current new reports suggest that Japan is also making overtures to China, whose agricultural potential is enormous.

63 Josling, 'Emerging agricultural trade', pp. 18–19.

64 McMichael, Philip (1993) 'World food system restructuring under a GATT regime', in Frances Ufkes (ed.) 'The political geography of agricultural trade', special issue of *Political Geography*, vol. 12, no. 3.

65 Gilmore, *A Poor Harvest*, p. 77.

66 In 1993, Canada, whose resources are fewer than those of the US, has refused to ship more subsidized grain to Russia despite the desperate state of the farm sector and the trade balance.

67 See McMichael, 'World food system restructuring'.

68 Homem de Melo, Fernando (1986) 'Unbalanced technological change and income disparity in a semi-open economy', in F. L. Tullis and W. L. Hollist (eds) *Food, State, and International Political Economy*, Lincoln, NB, University of Nebraska Press.

69 Jane Collins gives a remarkable account of the innovative labour relations and other practices of fruit and vegetable firms established in the wake of irrigation in the 1970s of the Sao Francisco Valley in North-eastern Brazil. See Collins, J. (1992) 'Production relations in irrigated agriculture – fruits and vegetables in the Sao Francisco Valley (Pernambuco/Bahia), Brazil', Working Paper No. 23,

Fresh Fruit & Vegetable Globalization Network, University of California, Santa Cruz. The Network has already produced a large number of working papers from its first conference, organized by William H. Friedland and David Goodman. Little has been published on this important aspect of global agro-food restructuring. For a news report on recent events in Brazil, see *Manchester Guardian Weekly*, 8 November 1992, p. 10.

70 Walton, John (1989) 'Debt, protest, and the state in Latin America', in Susan Eckstein (ed.) *Power and Popular Protest*, Berkeley, University of California Press.

71 For the general shift to corporate control in the 'new issues' of the Uruguay Round – services, intellectual property rights (TRIPs) and international investment rights (TRIMs) – see Majlof, Luis Abugattas (1991) 'World economic restructuring and the multilateral trade negotiations: the "new issues" in the Uruguay Round, problems and prospects for Latin America', Lincoln, NB, International Political Science Association. Also see Raghavan, Chakravarthi (1990) *Recolonization: GATT, the Uruguay Round and the Third World*, London, Zed Press. For agro-food corporations, see McMichael, P. 'GATT, global regulation, and the construction of a new hegemonic order', MS, Cornell University, 1992, and 'World food system restructuring'.

72 For the issue of genetic resources, see Kloppenberg, Jack (ed.) (1988) *Seeds and Sovereignty: the use and control of plant genetic resources*, Durham, NC and London, Duke University Press. For an instance of challenges to craft and regional products, France and the US disagree about the rules governing the names of wines, and this and related disputes reach to other countries and other products. Warren Moran (1993) has a fascinating discussion of the dispute over 'appellation contrôlée' in 'Rural space as intellectual property', in Ufkes (ed.) 'Political Geography'.

73 Already in 1976, J.-P. Berlan, J.-P. Bertrand and L. Lebas noted that 'les intérêts des agriculteurs et des multinationales américaines ne sont pas aussi unis que dans la période précédente'. See 'Eléments sur le développement du "complexe soja" américain dans le monde', *Revue Tiers-Monde* XVII, 66.

74 The details in each case can be found in Gilmore, *A Poor Harvest.*

75 Ibid., pp. 61–3.

76 For an excellent analysis of the long-term phenomenon, written before the current fluidity in the use of products for human and animal consumption became apparent, see Barkin, David, Batt, Rosemary L. and DeWalt, Billie (1990) *Food Crops vs. Feed Crops: global substitution of grains in production*, Boulder, CO and London, Lynne Rienner Publishers.

77 Byman, W. Jos (1990) 'New technologies in the agro-food system and US–EC trade relations', in P. Lowe, T. Marsden and S. Whatmore (eds) *Technological Change and the Rural Environment*, London, David Fulton, p. 148.

78 Raynolds, Laura (forthcoming) 'The restructuring of export agriculture in the Dominican Republic', and Friedland, William H. (forthcoming) 'The global fresh fruit and vegetable system', in McMichael, (ed.) *Global Restructuring.*

79 Ufkes, Frances 'The changing social structures of livestock marketing in Illinois, 1950–1990', MS, Association of American Geographers, Miami, April 1991 and Stanley, Kathleen (forthcoming) 'Industrial change and the transformation of rural labor markets in the US meatpacking industry', in McMichael (ed.) *Global Restructuring.*

80 Lawrence and Vanclay, 'Agricultural change and environmental degradation'.
81 Sanderson, Steven (1986) 'The emergence of the "World Steer": internationalization and foreign domination in Latin American cattle production', in F. L. Tullis and W. L. Hollist (eds) *Food, the State, and International Political Economy*, Lincoln, NB, University of Nebraska Press.
82 Byman, 'New technologies in the agro-food system', p. 148.
83 I have in mind examples from northern Italy, Mexico City and Toronto. For a discussion of the London Food Commission, created by the Greater London Council, see Jenkins, Robin (1990) 'Urban consumptionism as a route to rural renewal', in Bernstein et al. (eds) *The Food Question*.
84 These were the elements of the food policy adopted by the Swedish Social Democratic Party under electoral pressure from the Green Party in 1987. A supporting element was public education in the merits of locally produced foods, using lower chemical inputs and lower density of land use for grazing animals. All is suspended since the Swedish application to join the EC. See Vail, David (1991) 'Economic and ecological crises: transforming Swedish agricultural policy', in Friedland et al. (eds) *Towards a New Political Economy*.
85 For an analysis of the last extension of CONASUPO (Compania Nacional de Subsistencias Populares, or National Staple Products Company) into direct provision of food, shoes and other agro-food products in the Echeverria Administration, see Grindle, Merilee Serrill (1977) *Bureaucrats, Politicians and Peasants in Mexico*, Berkeley, University of California Press. It is possible to appreciate the merits, actual and potential, of the system without celebrating Mexican politics and bureaucracy.
86 For the connection between international regulation and regional agriculture, see Peterson, 'Paradigmatic shift'.
87 Philip McMichael and David Myhre, in 'Global regulation vs. the nation-state: agro-food restructuring and the new politics of capital', *Capital and Class* 43, 1991, argue for the possibility of a 'transnational state', consisting of strengthened ministries of trade and finance, integrated with each other and with international agencies, and distanced from other – especially social – national ministries. Robert Cox suggests a similar concept in *Production, Power and World Order*, New York, Columbia University Press, 1987.

11

International Law and the Right to Food

Philip Alston

Whether one speaks of human rights or basic human needs, the right to food is the most basic of all. Unless that right is first fulfilled, the protection of other human rights becomes a mockery for those who must spend all their energy merely to maintain life itself. . . . Unless all governments begin now to act upon their rhetorical commitments to ending hunger, the principle that human life is sacred, which forms the very underpinnings of human society, will gradually but relentlessly erode.

Presidential Commission on World Hunger, 1980

Introduction

Few human rights have been endorsed with such frequency, unanimity or urgency as the right to food, yet probably no other human right has been as comprehensively and systematically violated on such a wide scale in recent decades. The importance of the relevant norms in international law is attested to by the fact that the right to freedom from hunger is the only human right which the framers of the two International Human Rights Covenants specifically termed 'fundamental'. In addition, the right to food has been solemnly proclaimed by a succession of international conferences, in national constitutions, by governments and legislatures of all persuasions, and by many eminent and influential groups and individuals. Yet despite this impressive array of support for the right to food, no concerted effort has been made either to spell out in detail the implications of the relevant norm or to establish effective national and international machinery to promote compliance with existing international human rights obligations relating to food. While there is no shortage of reasons which have been proffered to justify this neglect, the magnitude of the continuing problems of hunger and malnutrition in the world demands that urgent consideration be given to proposals which might help to bridge the gap between the rhetoric and reality and thereby contribute to realization of the right to food.

Arguments Against Recognition of the Right to Food

Before looking at the existing international legal standards in this field, it is useful to take note of the main arguments that have been used to justify the international community's failure to undertake any meaningful codification of norms relating to the right to food.

The first argument is, in essence, that such an exercise would be a waste of time since moral and humanitarian considerations alone will not move governments or other relevant actors to respect the right to food. In this view food is first and foremost a commodity which is traded annually for billions of dollars and its status as a human right is very much secondary to this fact. A sympathetic version of this 'realist' thesis has been explained in the following terms by Haverberg:

> In theory, moral considerations should play a significant role in policy decisions. In practice, however, such factors *per se* are not taken into account at the national planning level. . . . Nutrition cannot be sold to governments on humanitarian grounds. Since moral dicta and nutritional principles generally converge, the most that can be hoped for is that nutritional considerations will play a more dominant role in policy formulation, and thus moral issues while not explicitly addressed will be implicitly implied.[1]

The second argument is that the complexity of the issues involved in promoting realization of the right, and the absence of a universal consensus on either the causes of, or the solutions to, the problem, make it virtually impossible to establish effective machinery for implementation of the right to food. Thus, in the personal view of the Legal Counsel to the Food and Agriculture Organization (FAO), J. P. Dobbert, the right to food 'is not enforceable at the international level and only within very narrow contractual limits at the national level'.

The third argument, which is generally applied to economic, social and cultural human rights as a whole, is that civil and political rights are of prior importance and that economic rights such as the right to food are only likely to be realized once freedom has been attained by the peoples of the world.

Existing International Legal Standards Relating to the Right to Food

There is a range of right-to-food-related standards which have been adopted to date as part of international treaty law. Article 25(1) of the Universal

Declaration of Human Rights of 1948 provides that 'everyone has the right to a standard of living adequate for the health and well-being of himself and his family, including food'. Any analysis of the most important legal source, article 11 of the International Covenant on Economic, Social and Cultural Rights, the ESCR Covenant, should be seen not only against the background of that provision, but also of several other articles of the Universal Declaration. The most important of these are: (1) article 3 which provides that 'everyone has the right to life'; (2) article 22 relating to the realization, through national efforts and international co-operation of economic, social and cultural rights; (3) article 28 which provides that 'everyone is entitled to a social and international order in which the rights and freedoms set forth in this Declaration can be fully realized'; and (4) article 29(1) which states that 'everyone has duties to the community'.

The right to self-determination which is the first article in each of the two Covenants, is sometimes mistakenly neglected in the context of the right to food. It is clear that there is a strong incentive for states which are genuinely committed to achieving and maintaining their right to self-determination to ensure food self-reliance. In addition, however, it is also arguable that a government would be in violation of the right to self-determination if it permitted the exploitation of the country's food-producing capacity (natural resources) in the exclusive interests of a small part of the population or of foreign (public or private) corporate interests while a large number of the state's inhabitants were starving or malnourished.

Article 6 of the International Covenant on Civil and Political Rights, which proclaims every human being's 'inherent right to life', is also relevant to the right to food. This point was underlined in 1982 by the Human Rights Committee which was established to supervise states' compliance with their obligations under that Covenant. The Committee observed that the expression 'inherent right to life' could not properly be interpreted in a restrictive manner and that protection of the right requires states to adopt positive measures rather than merely refraining from certain proscribed measures. More specifically, the Committee considered that it would be desirable for states parties to the Covenant 'to take all possible measures to reduce infant mortality and to increase life expectancy, especially in adopting measures to eliminate malnutrition and epidemics'.

Another important source in international law of guarantees of the right to food is to be found in the four Geneva Conventions of 1949 and their two Protocols of 1977. These instruments constitute the essence of modern international humanitarian law and they contain a number of provisions designed to ensure enjoyment of the right to food by both civilians and former combatants in time of war. Paradoxically, the relevant provisions are, in a number of respects, more detailed and comprehensive than those provisions of international law which govern realization of the right to food in peacetime.

None of the regional human rights instruments (the European Charter on Human Rights, the American Convention on Human Rights and the African Charter of Human and Peoples' Rights) contain any specific mention of the right to food. It appears that, in each case, the right to work and the right to social security are considered to be sufficiently comprehensive and to render specific provisions relating to food superfluous. The validity of this assumption would, however, appear to be questionable.

Article 11 of the ESCR Covenant

Article 11 of the International Covenant on Economic, Social and Cultural Rights proclaims the right to adequate food as well as the right to be free from hunger. Its pre-eminence among international right-to-food norms is due to the following factors: it represents a codification of the earlier norm contained in the Universal Declaration of Human Rights; its content was significantly shaped by the FAO; it is more detailed and specific than most other relevant international legal norms; 74 states (as at 1 September 1982) have formally accepted the obligation in international law to take steps to achieve progressively the full realization of the right; and a mechanism has been established under the Covenant to monitor states parties' compliance with their obligations, including those relating to the right to food.

Article 11 of the Covenant states as follows:

> 1. The States Parties to the present Covenant recognize the right of everyone to an adequate standard of living for himself and his family, including adequate food, clothing and housing, and to the continuous improvement of living conditions. The States Parties will take appropriate steps to ensure the realization of this right, recognizing to this effect the essential importance of international co-operation based on free consent.
> 2. The States Parties to the present Covenant, recognizing the fundamental right of everyone to be free from hunger, shall take, individually and through international co-operation, the measures, including specific programmes, which are needed:
> (a) To improve methods of production, conservation and distribution of food by making full use of technical and scientific knowledge, by disseminating knowledge of the principles of nutrition and by developing or reforming agrarian systems in such a way as to achieve the most efficient development and utilization of natural resources;
> (b) Taking into account the problems of both food-importing and food-exporting countries, to ensure an equitable distribution of world food supplies in relation to need.

Article 11 was drafted in response to a specific proposal by FAO. Debate on the article in the Third Committee of the General Assembly was relatively brief and it could be said that the wording of the proposed article was subjected to less demanding analysis and scrutiny than that of almost any other article in the Covenant.

In order to make effective use of any norm of international human rights law it is necessary to establish: its content; the subjects or beneficiaries; the objects or duty-holders; and mechanisms to promote compliance. Here, the first three of these aspects will be examined with respect to article 11 of the Covenant.

The Content of the Norm

The 'right to food' is in fact a shorthand expression encompassing two separate norms contained in article 11. The first, stated in paragraph 1, derives from the 'right of everyone to an adequate standard of living for himself and his family, including adequate food' and can be termed the right to adequate food. The second, proclaimed in paragraph 2, is the 'right of everyone to be free from hunger'. In most analyses that have been undertaken to date the two have been treated as being synonymous, with a preference nevertheless being shown for the latter. It is submitted that, while on the one hand there is a significant difference between the two norms, with the first being much broader than the second, on the other hand the term 'right to adequate food' is the appropriate overall one since there is no indication that paragraph 2 was intended by the drafters or by states which have ratified the Covenant to restrict or narrow the scope of the right proclaimed in paragraph 1.

The practical implications of taking, as the primary norm, the right to adequate food rather than the right to be free from hunger are significant. Whereas the former facilitates the adoption of a maximalist approach, the latter is able at least in theory to be satisfied by the adoption of policies designed to provide a minimum daily nutritional intake. While it may be appropriate to focus on freedom from hunger as a means by which to mobilize public support and as a starting point for national and international efforts, such an approach should be seen only as the first step towards realization of the primary norm which is the right to adequate food. In terms of quantity the notion of adequacy implies enough food to facilitate a normal, active existence rather than a minimum calorific package which does no more than prevent death by starvation. Moreover, in terms of quality the adequacy standard goes further than the freedom from hunger sub-norm in focusing on the cultural appropriateness of the food.

The principal objectives specified in article 11(2)(a), which deals with the national dimension of the right to food, are: to improve methods of food *production*; to improve methods of food *conservation*; and to improve methods of food *distribution*, all three with a view to promoting the realization of the right to food. In addition, the article lists other complementary objectives. They are: making full use of technical and scientific knowledge; disseminating knowledge of the principles of nutrition; and developing or reforming agrarian systems.

Two points about article 11(2)(a) warrant particular emphasis. The first is that none of the individual objectives is relevant for its own sake but only in so far as it contributes to the realization of the overall normative end, which is ensuring the right of everyone to be free from hunger. Thus, for example, the Covenant cannot be interpreted as supporting increased food production or agrarian reform *per se*. This fundamental point has all too often been neglected or even contradicted in analyses to date of the right to food. The second point is that attempts to distil from article 11(2)(a) an ordered, detailed, operational approach to the right to food are misplaced given the lack of detail and the degree of confusion which characterize the provision.

Nevertheless, the broad content of the norm is relatively clear and, taken as it is, it is sufficient to enable a determination in some cases that particular acts, or omissions to act, are either in conformity or in conflict with the norm. But this is clearly not enough if the right to food is to be fully implemented. The question then is whether anything has been done to elaborate upon the provisions of the basic norm. Two possibilities warrant examination in this regard. The first is whether instruments adopted by various organs since the adoption of the Covenant in 1966 can be considered to have contributed to a codification of the norm. The most prominent candidate would be the Universal Declaration on the Eradication of Hunger and Malnutrition adopted by the World Food Conference and endorsed by the General Assembly in 1974. Yet while the Declaration does proclaim the 'right to be free from hunger and malnutrition' it does not refer specifically either to article 25 of the Universal Declaration of Human Rights or to the Covenant. There is thus no stated intention of elaborating upon or interpreting the relevant provisions of the Covenant, and the content of the Declaration or similar instruments cannot be taken to constitute an authoritative interpretation of the norm.

The second potential means by which light could have been shed on the content of the norm is through the jurisprudence of the body charged with the supervision of states' compliance with their obligations under the Covenant. In practice, however, the Working Group established by the Economic and Social Council to assist it in this task has achieved nothing of any consequence in this respect.

The Subjects and Beneficiaries of the Right to Food

The principal holders of the right to food under the terms of article 11 are individuals. The right of individuals is formulated in terms of 'the right of everyone'. Whereas sub-paragraph 2 uses only this phrase, the terminology used in sub-paragraph 1 is 'the right of everyone . . . for himself and his family'. The question which then arises is to what exactly is the individual entitled? In practical terms, the answer will depend on the circumstances of the individual and of his or her geographical location at a given time. The most important point is to recognize the need to develop, at the national level, a set of relevant legal norms which reflects and seeks to satisfy the state's international legal obligation to promote the realization of the right of everyone to adequate food.

Another level at which one can identify a holder of the right to food is that of the state. Whether this is a collective right attaching directly to peoples or to states or whether it is rather an aggregation of the human rights of individuals which is articulated through the medium of the state, is an important theoretical question, but it is of limited practical relevance in the present context.

Article 11 does not specifically identify states as holders of the right to food. Nevertheless, by imposing duties upon states to act, 'through international co-operation', the article implicitly vests rights in certain states as a corollary of the duty of all states to act. Moreover, in practical terms, the obligation of states parties 'to ensure an equitable distribution of world food supplies in relation to need' can only be operationalized on an inter-state basis. The shield (or the sword) of state sovereignty severely restricts the possibility of implementing such an obligation at any other level.

The question of which states might be entitled to make claims on the grounds that they are subjects of the right to food, can only be answered on the basis of an assessment of the overall availability of food at the national level by comparison with the aggregated needs of the state's inhabitants for adequate food. The closest the international community has come to making such a global assessment is the category of 'most seriously affected countries' which were those which, in the wake of the 1972 oil-price rises, were deemed to be in need of emergency assistance to pay for minimum import requirements of food, fertilizers and industrial inputs. This categorization is effectively obsolete today. Other criteria would therefore need to be established in order to assess whether or not a particular country enjoys an equitable share of world food supplies in relation to need.

The Object or Duty-holders of the Norm

In analysing the duties relating to the right to food which derive from the relevant provisions of the Covenant, four main categories can be distinguished (UN 1980). They are: (1) states in respect of their domestic duties; (2) states in respect of their external duties; (3) individuals; and (4) the international community.

Before seeking to establish the scope and nature of these duties, it is useful to refer briefly to the approach to duties proposed by Henry Shue in his important work, *Basic Rights*.[2] He suggests that three types of duties correlate with every basic right. As applied to what he terms a 'subsistence right' such as the right to food, these are:

1 Duties not to eliminate a person's only available means of subsistence – duties to *avoid* depriving.
2 Duties to protect people against deprivation of the only available means of subsistence by other people – duties to *protect* from deprivation.
3 Duties to provide for the subsistence of those unable to provide for their own – duties to *aid* the deprived.

It is beyond the scope of this chapter to analyse the consequences for various entities of applying such an approach to the duties which attach to the right to food. Nevertheless, such an analysis will have to be undertaken sooner or later if the duties attaching to the right to food are to be spelt out and an appropriate system of accountability established. Such a system is an indispensable component of a comprehensive, balanced, practical and effective approach to the right to food.

States' domestic duties

In essence the domestic obligation of a state party to the Covenant is to take steps, to the maximum of its available resources with a view to achieving progressively the full realization of the right of everyone, without discrimination, to adequate food. A state party is also obliged to ensure that its own people is not in any case deprived of its own means of subsistence (article 1(2)) which must, as a minimum, be interpreted to include food.

The key issue as regards states parties' domestic duties concerns the meaning of the obligation 'to take steps'. It is clear (on the basis of the text both of article 2 and of articles 6–15 dealing with individual rights) that the phrase 'to the maximum of its available resources' should not lead to the obligation being viewed exclusively as a matter of making appropriate budgetary allocations. It is reasonable to assume on the basis of the practice of states in their reports under the Covenant that the 'steps' required to be taken include the adoption of some type of legislative, executive and/or administrative measures oriented specifically towards realization of the right in question. The validity of such an emphasis on the role of law is also confirmed by the provisions of article 2(2) whereby states parties 'undertake to guarantee' the exercise of the relevant rights without discrimination on certain grounds, and by the provisions of article 3 by which states parties 'undertake to ensure the equal right of men and women to the enjoyment' of the relevant rights, and article 4 whereby limitations on the enjoyment of rights are restricted to those 'determined by law'. In addition, article 11(1) commits states parties to 'take appropriate steps to *ensure* the realization of this right'.

In so far as a requirement to take legal or administrative measures can be deduced from the Covenant it does not amount to an obligation to ensure immediate realization. This is made abundantly clear by the use of the phrase 'achieving progressively'. Nevertheless, the leeway provided by this provision does not obviate the need to adopt at least rudimentary laws, and for regulations and/or policy statements designed to establish appropriate policies and to form the basis on which progressive realization can be built. As an indication of good faith this could be expected to include the drawing up of a coherent and, as far as possible, comprehensive plan setting out the steps to be followed in seeking to realize progressively the right to food.

In contrast to states parties' obligations under the Civil and Political Rights Covenant, states parties to the other Covenant are not required to ensure that an effective remedy is available to any person whose economic rights, including the right to food, are violated. This would not of course preclude the adoption of such an approach in domestic law or in the context of a regional human rights arrangement.

Thus, despite the apparent vagueness of the domestic duties of states to implement the Covenant's provisions on the right to food, their importance should not be underestimated. In addition to representing an international obligation on the basis of which they can be held accountable, politically as well as legally, states parties have also made a formal commitment against which their own peoples may assess their domestic policies.

States' external duties

General Assembly resolutions 34/46, 35/179 and 36/133 have recognized that

> in order fully to guarantee human rights and complete personal dignity, it is necessary to guarantee the right to (*inter alia*) . . . proper nourishment, through the adoption of measures at the national and international levels, including the establishment of the new international economic order.

This emphasis on the international dimensions of the right to food accurately reflects the approach adopted in the Covenant.

With respect to external duties states parties to the Covenant are obliged to take steps through international assistance and co-operation, especially economic and technical, to the maximum of their available resources with a view to achieving progressively the full realization of the right to food (article 2(1) and article 11). States are also required to avoid depriving any people of its own means of subsistence (article 1(2)). The 'essential importance of international co-operation' is further recognized in article 11(1), but it is stated to be 'based on free consent'. The significance of this qualification is open to debate. The qualification was presumably inserted as a safety clause against any assumption that food-surplus states have an automatic responsibility to make transfers to food-deficit states. Nevertheless, 'free consent' cannot reasonably be interpreted as nullifying the commitment to international co-operation by rendering it entirely optional. Nor can it defeat the overall responsibility provided for in article 2. It should thus be taken as meaning that while an obligation to international co-operation exists, the form which such co-operation will take is to be determined in accordance with the free consent of the state concerned.

States parties to the Covenant also undertake to take measures 'to ensure an equitable distribution of world food supplies in relation to need' and in so doing to take 'into account the problems of both food-importing and food-exporting countries' (article 11(2)(b)).

By applying the approach proposed by Henry Shue, it is possible, in general terms, to arrive at the following list of duties which could be derived from this obligation.

A *Duties to avoid depriving*

1 The duty to avoid international policies and practices which deprive other states of their means of subsistence or which promote an inequitable distribution of world food supplies.

2 The duty to mitigate national policies which have the effect of promoting an inequitable distribution of world food supplies.

3 The duty not to use food as an international sanction (discussed below).

B *Duties to protect from deprivation*

4 The duty to ensure that international trade and aid policies and practices contribute as far as possible to the equitable distribution of world food supplies.

5 The duty to regulate the activities of domestically based entities (including transnational corporations and state trading enterprises) whose activities have, or might have, a significant impact on the distribution of world food supplies.

C *Duties to aid the deprived*

6 The duty of food-surplus states to contribute to emergency buffer schemes and to assist in cases of internationally declared emergencies.

7 The duty to co-operate as far as possible with multilateral programmes which are aimed at ensuring an equitable distribution of world food supplies.

It is clear, however, that such a list of duties is of limited practical value in the short term. What is required in the longer term is the transformation of these duties into a legally binding instrument which is presented as an elaboration of the general obligation laid out in article 11.

The duties of individuals

Before considering the question of the individual's duty to promote regulation of the right to food, it must be noted that in human rights debates at the international level relatively little attention has been given to the overall question of the specific duties which may be considered to correlate to the rights spelt out in the international Bill of Human Rights. In general terms, however, the Preamble to each of the Covenants states that the individual does have 'duties to other individuals and to the community to which he belongs [and] is under a responsibility to strive for the promotion and observance of the rights recognized' in the Covenant. In the context of the right to food this would seem to involve, as a minimum, a duty not to overconsume and not to waste food.

The range of individual duties could of course be further expanded in line with Shue's categories discussed above. In practice, the important point is that states parties to the Covenant are not only entitled, but are required, to give careful consideration to measures designed to promote the observance, on the part of individuals, of their relevant duties with respect to the right to food.

The duties of the international community

The duty to co-operate internationally is affirmed in general terms in articles 55 and 56 of the UN Charter and specifically in terms of the right to food in article 11 in conjunction with article 2 of the Covenant. To a large extent the duties which can be attributed to the international community on the basis of the Covenant have been discussed above in relation to states' external duties. Further consideration, however, needs to be given to the duties relating to the right to food which can be attributed to the various food policies and operational agencies established by the international community. It is clear, however, that the various agencies themselves should be encouraged to undertake in-depth analyses of their own obligations as regards the right to food.

Conclusion

This survey of issues raised by the right to food provision of article 11 of the ESCR Covenant does not provide us with a particularly encouraging picture. Rather, it shows that, while the basic norm is clearly enunciated, no amount of strict legal construction or interpretation of the subsidiary norms will suffice to produce a clear and widely acceptable framework within which the right to food could be effectively operationalized. A convention spelling out the normative implications of the right to food is thus a fundamental prerequisite to effective action by states and by the international community towards operationalization of the right to food. Until such an exercise is undertaken, the concept of a right to food as a human right will continue to be abused for rhetorical purposes while being ignored for all practical purposes.

NOTES

1 Haverbeg, L. (1977) 'Individual needs: nutritional guidelines for policy?', in L. Brown and H. Shue (eds) *Food Policy: the responsibility of the United States in the life and death choices*, New York, Free Press, p. 212.
2 Shue, Henry (1980) *Basic Rights: subsistence, affluence and U.S. foreign policy*, Princeton, NJ, Princeton University Press, p. 53.

FURTHER READING

Brownlie, I. (1987) *The Human Right to Food*, London, Commonwealth Secretariat.
Eide, A. (1989) *Right to Adequate Food as a Human Right*, Human Rights Study Series No. 1, New York, United Nations.
Hilf, M. (1987) 'The right to food in national and international law', in T. Oppermann and E. U. Petersmann (eds) *Reforming the International Economic Order*, Berlin, Duncker and Humblot, pp. 125–46.
Robertson, R. E. (1989–90) 'The right to food – Canada's broken covenant', *Canadian Human Rights Year Book*, Toronto, Carswell, pp. 185–216.
Saxena, J. N. (1990) 'The right to food', *Delhi Law Review* 12, 126–32.

12

Hunger, Needs and Rights

Onora O'Neill

In the 1990s, there are hundreds of millions of human beings who go hungry. At most times, there are millions whose hunger is so severe that they starve, become ill and may die. Where there is famine, many starve. The publicity given to these events often suggests that hunger and famine are natural disasters, produced by floods, droughts, blight and other forces of nature. However, it is increasingly clear that bad weather and pests alone need not and do not produce massive human disasters. Weather and pests do so only when social and economic structures are too fragile to cope with normal fluctuations. Where social and economic structures are robust enough to provide for harsh climates and other recurrent difficulties we do not accept high death rates as natural. Nobody would accept the deaths of many southern Californians because they live in a natural desert or of Minnesotans because of severe winters. The problems of hunger and famine in other parts of the world are also not irremediable natural realities.

Given that these disasters are remediable, we can raise many practical questions about them. The questions most often asked are 'how' questions. How can hunger be reduced? Is it a matter of advances in agriculture? Of higher investment in poor economies? Of reducing population growth? Of reforming systems of land tenure? Of preventing migration to the cities? Of massive transfer of resources from rich to poor countries? These questions are complicated; probably different answers are needed for different situations and different parts of the world.

Before we reach the 'how' questions, however, we must answer certain 'why' questions. Why should we take steps to deal with world hunger? Is world hunger perhaps a problem for those who are hungry, but of no concern to those of us who have enough to eat? What claims have the hungry on us? Is it wrong to do nothing? Why? If we come to the conclusion that there is nothing wrong with leaving the hungry to starve, then there is little reason to ask 'how' questions. This chapter will look at some of the ways in which we might approach the 'why' questions. If we find that there are good reasons to help the hungry, we will not have 'the answers', but we at least will have reason for putting energy and resources into answering the 'how' questions.

Needs and Happiness

Imagine that your doorbell rings one evening and you find on the doorstep an emaciated family. They obviously are hungry and desperate. Few of us would hesitate. We are clear enough about the urgency of need when it is in front of our eyes. Of course, we might not have enough food, or we might hope to hand the problem over to welfare officials quickly; but for most of us the thought of turning a starving person from our homes is repugnant. In Christian and Jewish thought, and in other religious traditions also, meeting others' *needs*, including the needs of strangers, is and has always been a central matter of ethical concern and refusal to help those in great need is seen as a paradigm of wrongdoing.

Yet when we turn to present-day ethical theories, we find that need is often no longer a central category. This transformation of popular and philosophical ethical thinking has taken various forms, of which utilitarian reasoning and human rights theories are probably the most significant today, at least in the English-speaking world.

Utilitarian thinking concentrates on seeking those optimal lines of action that will secure the greatest total happiness. Of course, meeting needs is often one way of producing happiness, but it is not the only way, and for utilitarians, meeting needs has no automatic priority over other ways of making people happy. If maximal happiness were produced by action that leaves some people in need – or even exacerbates their needs – then, according to utilitarian thinking, it would be wrong to meet those needs.

This harsh conclusion is often blurred. Sometimes meeting needs will maximize happiness; sometimes it is quite unclear which line of action would maximize happiness. Utilitarian writers disagree about which policies are optimal. Some hold that a massive transfer of resources from rich to poor will maximize happiness. These theorists suggest (invoking standard marginalist considerations) that a given sum of money or other resources yields more happiness for those who start with less. But other utilitarian thinkers have reasoned that transfer payments will produce economic dependence and (they suggest) fuel population growth, which ultimately outstrips all possible aid and so will lead to dire misery in the long run.[1] According to this view, maximal happiness would be produced by leaving those in greatest need to suffer the consequences. Even if utilitarians could settle their disputes, they would still be committed to the production of happiness rather than the alleviation of need. All utilitarian thinking sets as much store by increasing the happiness of somebody who is in no way needy as by equivalent increases of happiness produced by meeting needs.

Utilitarianism is a mode of ethical thinking that takes a subjective view of what is good. What matters is happiness, the experiences that we subjectively have. Thinking about human needs is a matter of thinking about what is objectively required for fulfilled human life. Sometimes people want and would be made happy by things that stand in the way of their needs being met. They may want cigarettes more than good health or their traditional way of life more than a modern one that reduces poverty or increases food supplies.

Here we begin to see some of the deeper reasons why the category of need has faded from modern ethical thought. We hesitate to declare that we can know what is objectively good. We have lost the certainties of classical and of religious ethics about what human beings need in order to lead good and flourishing lives. If we cannot be sure what the good is, how can we claim that human beings need certain things and that meeting their needs should take priority over the pursuit of happiness? The category of need became marginal in modern ethical thinking with the rejection of the Aristotelian and Christian picture of a determinate human nature, whose flourishing or fulfilment would be thwarted if certain conditions – those that humans need – were not met. In its place much modern political and ethical thought placed the pursuit of happiness. Indeed, much modern liberal thinking claims to be 'agnostic about the good for man'.[2]

Needs and Rights

Utilitarian thinking is not the only modern approach to ethical issues in which the category of need has become marginal. Theories of human rights, which became immensely influential in the last 20 years, also place little weight on meeting human needs. What does it take to show that people have some right? One necessary requirement is surely to show that others have obligations to respect or fulfil that right. If nobody has such obligations, there just is no right at all. There cannot be a right not to be assaulted unless others have an obligation not to assault. There cannot be a right to vote unless others have an obligation not to interfere with voting. You have no right to the bank paying out the money you have deposited unless the bank has an obligation to do so. This is commonplace and uncontroversial. So we could begin the task of showing that everybody has a right to food by showing that there is a counterpart obligation to provide that food to which everybody has a right. Here we find a major obstacle.

We have a right if we are entitled to claim certain sorts of action or forbearance from whomever holds the counterpart obligation. There is a right to food only if there is some agent or institution that has the obligation to provide food to those who are hungry. Who has such an obligation? We can imagine a wide variety of answers. For example, the obligation to feed the hungry belongs to their own families or communities; to the government of the country in which they live; to the United Nations or to other corporate, voluntary or political international organizations; or to the citizens of more prosperous parts of the world. Usually when people are really hungry it is pointless to suggest that their families or local communities have an obligation to provide food. Real hunger occurs precisely when local resources are exhausted. However, who else has the obligation? Unless we can answer this question, asserting that there is a right to food or a right to have one's basic needs met is mere, and callous, rhetoric.

Two conflicting answers are currently given to this question by writers on human rights. One answer, the libertarian answer, is that nobody has an obligation to feed the hungry, and consequently the hungry have no right to food, unless they have entered into special relationships by which others incurred special obligations to feed them. The other answer, the welfare answer, contends that because there is a right to food (and to other necessities of life), every person and every political entity, including each nation-state, has obligations to make good on this right by assigning and then enforcing obligations to provide food for the hungry. These two visions of human rights have radically different implications for problems of world hunger. I shall sketch these before turning to the arguments that we might use for or against either vision.

Two Visions of the Rights of the Hungry

The libertarian vision of human rights sees all fundamental rights as *liberty rights* or freedoms from others' interference. Rights are simply entitlements not to be interfered with. Because needs cannot be met merely by a policy of non-interference, there can be no right to have one's needs met. The hungry have no right to food. The only way anybody can acquire a right to some positive action or service from another is when the two have entered some special relationship. For example, if somebody hungry has bought food, he or she is entitled to have it delivered and the vendor has an obligation to deliver; if somebody is a member of a family that has food supplies, he or she has the customary entitlements of relatives to share in the available food. Those who are really hungry usually lack special rights to food.

Within a libertarian vision of rights there is no required response to others' need, however dire. At the same time, libertarians often will remind those who criticize them as harsh or callous that they leave room for, and indeed admire, voluntary charitable action undertaken by individuals and that charity may save the hungry.

This appeal to charity is unconvincing for two reasons. The first reason is that as things are in the world today, hunger is far too large a problem, and far too closely connected with major issues of political and economic power and policy, to be remedied by individual voluntary action. Charity may help in the short run where there has been major political or economic failure, but charity cannot substitute for the sustained working of effective institutions and policies that prevent hunger. Even when nothing better can be offered in the short term, charity cannot substitute for good development policies.

The illusion that charity is the appropriate response to world hunger is sustained by comparisons made in the media (also in the publicity of major charities) between one-time emergencies, such as earthquakes, floods or wars, and long-term, systemic problems, such as world hunger. The comparison is apt in one way: like natural disasters and wars, world hunger causes hideous suffering and shortens lives. But in other ways the comparison is inept. Most hungry people have not suffered any sudden disruption or disaster that can be remedied by emergency relief. Alas, the hungry are mostly living their normal lives, with their normal resources and their ordinary social and economic relations, which are too fragile to sustain what are often quite minor ups and downs of climate, harvest or market forces. We all know that slight declines in supplies can trigger large price rises, create incentives to hoard, and leave the weakest unable to compete in the market. When the market we are talking about is the market for the means of life, these abstract economic forces end lives. Short-term relief of the sorts charities aim to organize can prevent immediate deaths, but cannot produce the social or economic transformations that sustain lives.

The second problem with relying on charity as a response to hunger or other major human needs is that charity is not taken seriously within the libertarian vision. Traditional religious views of charity saw it as a matter of obligation. Obligations of charity were not 'perfect' obligations, to which rights correspond; yet they were considered real, if 'imperfect' obligations. In the Western religious tradition, there was no suggestion that 'imperfect' obligations were optional. These obligations were called imperfect only to indicate that they were incomplete. Given that we cannot provide all help that is needed by all others on all occasions, our obligations to help meet needs must be incomplete in the sense that we cannot do everything and cannot (in the abstract) specify whom we should help when and how much. Because we cannot identify who among the possible recipients of help is entitled to help from which others, we cannot speak of rights to be helped. By contrast, obligations not to interfere can be complete – it is possible to refrain from battering, killing or defrauding *all* others at *all* times, so here we can talk of corresponding rights. In traditional views, help to the needy and justice are both obligatory, but justice can be accorded to all, while help can be given only to some. Hence, the allocation of justice assigns rights to the recipients, but the allocation of help does not.

It is an interesting intellectual, or perhaps ideological, curiosity of the present day that many people profess commitment to two incompatible ethical positions. Many advocate a libertarian vision of rights, which takes seriously only those obligations not to interfere that correspond to liberty rights. Yet the same people also claim to be committed to religious traditions that take a wider view of obligations and think it obligatory to help meet the needs of others, including the needs of strangers. *Laissez faire* is embraced together with the parable of the Good Samaritan. Those who are aware of the conflicts between these visions of human obligations sometimes try to resolve the conflicts by insisting that the libertarian vision is correct for public affairs and the religious vision for the private domain. There is a long chapter of Western intellectual history behind this attempted reconciliation of incompatibles. Although a discussion of this attempted reconciliation is beyond the scope of this chapter, I can point out some of the central questions such a discussion would have to raise. How should we distinguish between public and private spheres? If we relegate a religious vision to a private sphere and deny its application to matters public and political, are we taking the vision seriously? In particular, is an interpretation of the parable of the Good Samaritan that limits its applicability to private and local matters consonant with the actual message of the parable? Or does such a privatized interpretation tacitly subordinate the Christian vision to the libertarian one?

The second widely discussed contemporary vision of human rights also sees liberty rights as central human rights. Unlike the libertarian view, however, this second vision asserts that there are also rights to certain sorts of goods and services, and in particular to the fulfilment of basic needs. For example, some maintain that there are rights to food, rights to basic health care and rights to education. These rights are commonly referred to as welfare rights.[3]

But establishing that there are welfare rights has proved a difficult task. Appeal to grand international or constitutional documents is no more decisive here than it is for the libertarian vision of all rights as liberty rights. If we are to settle the debates about fundamental rights, we have to go beyond the charters and proclamations.

It hardly needs saying that it will matter a great deal to those who are hungry how this issue is decided. Behind the ebb and flow of current politics and economic struggles lie legal and institutional structures and policies whose form reflects (no doubt imperfectly) certain conceptions of human obligations. If we could show that our only obligations are to respect liberty rights, we could vindicate a *laissez-faire* policy toward the needs of the hungry. All that the poor and hungry would be owed are the same freedoms from interference that those with plenty are owed. If, on the other hand, we could establish that there are welfare as well as liberty rights, obligations would not be met and justice could not be achieved by institutions or policies that take a *laissez-faire* approach to others' needs. Justice to those in need might demand arduous and specific action on the part of those who have the obligations to meet those needs. It is no idle theoretical concern that leads us to consider the fundamental arguments offered by various theories of human rights. I shall look in turn at the prospects for establishing libertarian rights and a broader conception of human rights that includes welfare rights.

Libertarian Constructions of Rights

Libertarian thinking takes the notion of liberty as fundamental and interprets this liberty in a quite restricted way as a matter of freedom from interference. Human rights are defined as the set of arrangements needed to guarantee equal and maximal liberty for all. Modern interpretations of this thought are sophisticated and clear. Unlike the eighteenth-century documents, such as Tom Paine's *The Rights of Man* or the Declarations of Rights of the American and French Revolutions, present-day interpretations do not base rights on a mixture of appeals to self-evidence, human nature or divine authority. Contemporary theories of human rights try to justify a specific list of rights by constructing the set of rights that would constitute the best realization of equal liberty for all. Of course, some people doubt whether liberty, however interpreted, should be given this fundamental status. I propose to leave that issue aside and consider whether, if we accepted that liberty was fundamental, the libertarian construction would work. If the construction works, we then will need to check whether the platform on which it rests – the priority given to (a certain interpretation of) liberty – is sound. If the construction does not even work, we can spare ourselves that labour.

The construction of a libertarian account of human rights requires that we find the *largest* set of liberties that is *consistently extendable to everybody*.[4] It is easy to see how this standard can be used to rule out certain rights as spurious. Liberty rights are consistently extendable only when the counterpart obligations not to interfere are compatible with the exercise of the right. We can see that there can be no rights to privileges, or rights to success, or rights to win in competitive activities, for all these rights would require that others grant us privileges or successes that would prevent them having a like right. Such bogus rights could not in principle be held by all.

However, we cannot provide a libertarian construction of rights just by ruling out those spurious rights that cannot be extended to all. We also would have to show which one of many mutually consistent, universally extendable sets of rights should be preferred. This stage of the libertarian construction faces serious difficulties. There is no unique set of rights that includes all others. Because liberty rights can themselves be in conflict, we cannot construct a consistent set that includes all possible liberty rights. For example, there cannot be both an unconditional right of access to public places *and* an unconditional right of assembly in public places for political purposes. If both rights were unconditional, they would conflict with one another. Hence, one or the other of these possible rights must be excluded from any consistent set of rights. There are many ways in which rights of assembly and of access can be accommodated to one another. The same holds true for other sets of liberty rights. To determine which rights human beings actually have, we need to work out which set of mutually consistent, universally holdable rights is *largest*. Yet there is no ready way to do this, for there is no metric that tells us which rights or sets of rights are larger or more extensive than other rights or sets of rights.

Given this lack of metric, it is puzzling that rights theorists make such widespread use of the idea of the most extensive liberty. What creates the impression that we can tell which set of liberty rights is the largest? I believe that the impression is due in very large part to the constant use of a set of *spatial* or *territorial* and often *proprietary* metaphors in discussions of rights. Rights constantly are spoken of as 'spheres' or 'territories', which right-holders are entitled to defend by excluding others. Those who violate rights are said to 'invade' others' rights or to 'cross borders'.

These metaphors have a long history. They arose in seventeenth- and eighteenth-century Europe, whose central political concerns were the power and conflicts of nation-states and their territorial integrity, and whose economic development often centred on the enclosure of land whose use had once been either common or unassigned. In such a world, as well as in the New Worlds, where conquest and colonization, 'clearing' native peoples and establishing plantations, and homesteading, ranching and vanishing frontiers obtained, it was all too easy to think of all rights on the model of property rights and of property rights on the model of owning a piece of land – what came to be called 'a property'. This history encouraged the illusion that rights themselves, rather than some things that people (may) have (exclusive) rights to use, have spatial dimensions. Illusion it is, however. Even rights in landed property do not literally have size or shape. They are rights to use certain resources in certain ways to the exclusion of others. A right is not any larger when it is exercised over a larger area or object. Somebody who buys both a loaf of bread and a roll does not have a larger right to the loaf.

If rights do not literally have a spatial structure, we cannot determine which set of possible liberty rights is the greatest. Distinct rights can be made mutually consistent in varied, mutually exclusive ways; hence, we can find no all-encompassing set of rights. Nor is there even a core set of basic liberty rights that is included in all consistent sets of liberty rights. Consider any two putative members of such a core set of rights. They, too, could be mutually adjusted in varied ways, thereby forming alternative core sets and precluding any unique core set. Therefore, we cannot establish what human rights there are by looking for a largest consistent set of liberty rights.

This argument meets those who advocate a libertarian interpretation of rights on their chosen ground. The point is not that libertarians fail to pay enough attention to human needs and welfare, for libertarian advocates would retort that justice requires no attention to needs or welfare. Rather, libertarian accounts of justice fail in their chosen objective of providing an account of maximal liberty. Nevertheless, the critical argument advanced here does not provide us with an adequate account of human rights. The inadequacy of libertarian constructions does not show that other accounts of human rights succeed; it shows only that the libertarian construction of rights does not work.

Welfare Rights Constructions

An alternative approach to constructing a theory of rights is used by those who think that there are welfare as well as liberty rights. One promising line of argument is the following: rights of all sorts are of use and value only to those who can act. Even paradigmatic liberty rights, such as rights to vote or to speak freely, are useless to those who cannot act. Those who are starving, physically weak or abysmally ignorant cannot use such liberty rights. Hence, if there are *any* rights, there must be *basic rights* to have needs met. Basic rights are rights to those goods, services or liberties that are needed if human beings are to become and remain agents. Human agency fails to develop if children are starved or grossly deprived of socialization; hence, it would be a basic right that these needs be met. Human agency is destroyed by severe damage to health, by hunger and oppression; hence, it would be a basic right that needs for survival, including basic health, food and minimal physical security, be met. Some basic rights must be welfare rights.

This is an impressive line of reasoning that has been developed and refined by several recent writers[5] and is conceived of as a critique of the libertarian view of rights. This critique confronts anybody who already holds that there are rights with reasons to think that these must include welfare as well as liberty rights. It insists that human beings are not ideal, disembodied agents, but material beings whose agency depends on their material needs being met. However, those not already committed to thinking that there are human rights are given no reasons to conclude that there are. The argument, as sketched, might lead in either of two directions. We might conclude (1) that because there are rights there are also basic welfare rights or (2) that neither basic welfare nor other rights have been established.

What reason can those who hold the first view give for thinking that there are any rights? If these theorists are to be convincing, they must at least show who bears the obligations that are the counterpart to such rights. Advocates of a libertarian conception of justice have no difficulty in showing to whom the counterpart obligations are allocated. Because libertarians hold that all rights are liberty rights, the only recognized obligations are negative obligations not to interfere, which fall universally on all individuals and all institutions. The obligations that correspond to liberty rights can and must be universal obligations; liberty is curtailed if anybody or any institution is permitted to infringe it. But advocates of welfare rights cannot plausibly use this line of argument. The obligations that must exist if there are any welfare rights are obligations to provide goods and services to particular persons at particular places. It would be absurd to claim that everyone has an obligation to provide a morsel of food or a fraction of an income to each deprived person. Goods and services have to be rendered by particular persons or institutions to some others.

Advocates of welfare rights face the problem that allocation *cannot* here be universal and thus remains undetermined. Some have argued that this raises no problem once we address the institutionalization of rights.[6] All rights, even liberty rights, can be enforced only by allocating specific powers and obligations to particular agents and institutions. In this respect, there is nothing special about welfare rights. However, we cannot move on to questions of enforcement until we know what human rights there are. For we would not know what should be enforced.

There is a real asymmetry between welfare and liberty rights that cannot be overcome by postponing the question of who has obligations to meet whose basic needs and treating it as a matter that arises only in contexts of enforcing and institutionalizing rights. Yet we cannot simply assume that existing institutions (states? international agencies? transnational corporations? charities?) should meet welfare rights. First, current institutional structures may be sources of world hunger rather than of its remedy; hence, allocating obligations to meet needs on the basis of the status quo may backfire. Second, appeals to existing laws and institutions in the course of an argument to discover what rights there are only beg questions; such appeals commit what is often called the naturalistic fallacy.

The Perspective of Obligations

The project of constructing a determinate account of human rights looks unpromising. Even a libertarian theory of rights is indeterminate, and theories that include welfare rights face further difficulties in allocating the obligations that correspond to welfare rights. Yet if obligations are unallocated, we have no more than the rhetoric of charters and manifestos. In addition, theories that make rights fundamental are mute on the subject of imperfect obligations.

These two problems are closely linked. Imperfect obligations were supposed to be obligations to help and support others. If all ethical relations are grounded in rights and all rights are liberty rights, then imperfect obligations vanish. This is a point to which proponents of welfare rights are sensitive. These proponents take seriously the libertarian criticism that no rights correspond to imperfect obligations, which are therefore no matter of justice, and undertake to show that help and support to others in need is, after all, a matter of perfect obligation and therefore is as central to justice as the recognition of liberty rights. If the argument had succeeded, we would at least have less need for a theory of imperfect obligations; those in need would find in welfare rights better arguments for demanding others' help than they could have mustered within the terms of any theory of imperfect obligation.

However, if the argument for welfare rights also fails to allocate the corresponding obligations, our best strategy may be to stay within a conceptual framework that takes imperfect obligations seriously. This cannot be done within the framework of any theory that makes rights the fundamental ethical category because no rights correspond to imperfect obligations. However, by reversing our perspective we can reach a standpoint that affords a view of imperfect obligations. The alternative perspective can be explored by constructing a theory of obligations rather than of rights.

If we were able to construct a theory of obligations, the problem of the allocation of obligations would be solved in the process of construction, although it would still be the case that imperfect obligations lacked counterpart rights. This, however, might not be a practical disaster. Those who have obligations can seek to fulfil them whether or not particular others have rights to the performance of those obligations. Imperfect obligations can even be enforced, although their performance cannot be claimed by particular right-holders. (Of course, we may conclude that imperfect obligations ought not to be enforced, but that is a further question.) While rights without counterpart obligations are mere rhetoric, obligations without counterpart rights provide agents with solid reasons to act.

A change of perspective from rights to obligations makes agents and agency central. Theories of rights indeed see agents as indispensable (without agents, no rights could be recognized or respected), yet oddly focus on those who are to *receive* rather than on those who are to *act*. There are political and rhetorical reasons why this focus is sometimes useful. When the aim is to exert pressure from below to secure the performance of obligations that are not acknowledged, the best or only strategy may be to galvanize the powerless to claim others' action. Galvanizing may work best when the powerless see themselves as holders of rights. Yet no amount of galvanizing would have effect if the (relatively) powerful could not act, for pressure and encouragement could not then bring them to do so.

If we take a long view, we can see that the perspective of agents and their obligations, rather than that of right-holders and their entitlements, is not only conceptually more basic but has been historically more important. The notion of obligation has been part of all ethical and political thought, secular and religious, since antiquity. The notion of rights is a seventeenth-century innovation, and the notion that rights are ethically basic is an eighteenth-century one. Yet neither innovation gained new ground. Even an incomplete theory of obligations – the part that deals only with perfect obligations – provides all that is needed to ground rights; a more complete theory of obligations captures matters that must be ignored by those who make rights fundamental. Nothing then is lost by adopting the broader perspective of obligations, and something may be gained.

The Universalizing Construction

How could we construct a theory of human obligations? A first move might be the exact counterpart of the one used to construct theories of rights. We could begin by insisting that all should have the same fundamental obligations (whose specific requirements might vary with circumstance). This amounts only to denying that some are by nature privileged or by nature subordinate. If we are neither natural slaves nor natural masters, it is reasonable that we should have the same obligations. This thought can be expressed in a different way by aiming to construct *principles of obligation* that could hold for all human beings. Universal human obligations cannot be based on principles that presume privilege for some; an articulation of universal obligations must reject principles of action that cannot be shared by all.

By itself this may seem a slender basis for any theory of human obligations. Nevertheless, the insistence that human obligations require us to reject principles that cannot be acted on by all is not new. It is the very standard Immanuel Kant used in the late eighteenth century when he constructed the first account of human obligations that appealed neither to tradition nor to religion. Following Kant's lead we may label this method for constructing the outline of an account of human obligations a universalizing construction. Of course, venerable antecedents are no guarantee of sound argument; we had better move slowly in considering the possibility of constructing a theory of universal obligations. We can begin by rehearsing what it is to have an obligation.

When we have an obligation, we are required to do or omit some type of action. Sometimes we are required to do or omit this type of action for *all* others. Sometimes we are required to do or omit it for *specified* others. Sometimes we are required to do or omit the action for *unspecified* others, but not for *all* others. Obligations of the first two sorts – universal and special perfect obligations – may be thought of as having corresponding rights. Obligations of the third sort cannot plausibly be thought of as having corresponding rights; they are (whether universal or special) imperfect obligations. All of this is just a review of terrain we have explored, which is now mapped from the perspective of the agent rather than from the perspective of those entitled to receive action of a certain type from others.

What sorts of principles of action are ruled out by reliance on a universalizing construction? Can principles that are acted on by each be acted on by all? Will any exceptions that refer to unique achievements or particular objects be trivial? To be sure, not everyone can eat the same loaf or live in the same house. However, we do not expect principles of action to be peculiar to individual cases. Principles of action are presumably fairly indeterminate; they are formulated to apply to a range of cases, not to a unique or privileged situation. A universalizing construction of obligations demands not that any (or every) principle of action that uses some arbitrary description of a given act be universally adoptable, but that the fundamental principles that govern the choice of particular actions be so.[7]

Not every fundamental principle of action is universally adoptable. There are certain principles that can be acted on by any one person, but cannot be acted on by all. Consider the principle of deceiving (whose varied modes include fraud, false promising and cheating). Deceit only works against a background of trust; trust would be destroyed by universal deceit; hence, successful deceit requires that not everybody deceive. A principle of deceit cannot be universalized; the universalizing construction shows that it is a human obligation to avoid action that is based on principles of deceit.

An analogous argument shows that the rejection of principles of coercion is also a matter of obligations. Coercion, too, has many modes, which include the use of force, threat and, more specifically, slavery, torture and forced labour. Each mode of coercion denies or destroys the agency of its victims. This reveals that a principle of coercion cannot be universally acted on. Principles can be universally acted on only when others' agency is respected, and the core of respect for agency is not to destroy or override it.

These two arguments are closely connected to those by which libertarian thinkers establish human rights. Libertarian arguments also establish obligations that are universally held and are owed to all other agents. Non-coercion and non-deceit are generally a matter of not interfering with others' agency, either by circumventing it (deceit) or by overriding or destroying it (coercion). These are perfect obligations, matters of justice that are owed by all to all. In this domain, constructivist accounts of obligations are the mirror image of constructivist accounts of rights. Each construction is a demonstration that those who do not have ethical relations that reflect privilege and subordination have mutual rights and obligations that exclude destroying, coercing or deceiving one another.

These principles of obligation cast a severe light on the European penetration and annexation of other continents in the early modern period. Colonizers standardly did serious injustice to the native peoples whose lives they disrupted and ended and whose land they took. Deceit and coercion, even slavery, were the order of the day. From Connecticut to the Congo, genocide was frequent. Those of us who are descendants of the explorers and colonists can look back in shame.

We can also wonder how much rectification is owed for undoubted injustices. If those who did the wrongs and their victims were still alive, we would surely think that restitution and compensation were necessary and appropriate; they would be urgent matters of rectificatory justice, analogous to questions about punishment of Nazi war criminals and compensation for their victims. However, we are now by and large so distant from the crimes of colonialism that we cannot tell who ought to make what restitution to whom. So many victims have perished, often without descendants; so many crimes are unrecorded. We doubt whether the sins of the fathers should be visited on the children and often cannot identify the children. Perhaps some or much of the hunger of today can be traced in part to ancient wrongs; but too much is obscure for us to work out just what restitution and punishment are appropriate.

If ancient wrongs cannot now be righted, can we assume that we have met our obligations to those who are hungry provided we now refrain from deceit and coercion? Does the universalizing construction of obligations conform to the libertarian construction of perfect rights and demand no more than policies of national non-coercion and commercial *laissez faire*? Would such policies be enough to secure justice for the poverty-stricken parts of the world?

Laissez faire – non-interference – is hardly possible in an interdependent world. For *laissez faire* is not just a matter of refusing help to others, but of not interfering in their action in *any* way. The powerful nations and institutions that determine conditions of manufacture, credit and trade for the poor world do not practise *laissez faire*; these actors fix the conditions of life and survival for others.

The distance between the refusal of help that passes for *laissez faire* and genuine non-interference shows that the universalizing construction of obligations and the libertarian construction of rights are only superficially similar. The libertarian construction looks at what should be received and provides arguments for (supposedly) specific freedoms from interference. Here the emphasis is entirely on non-interference, and the reliance on spatial metaphors appears to allow a simple interpretation of non-interference as a matter of keeping out, of staying away, of doing nothing.

A constructivist account of obligations, by contrast, focuses on actions; it demands that action be based on universally adoptable principles, such as non-deceit and non-coercion. These standards cannot be satisfied merely by policies of selective *laissez faire*, such as neglect of others' needs. Genuine *laissez faire* would require complete severance of relations with others. The reality of what is dishonestly now called *laissez faire* is that powerful nations, institutions and individuals coerce and deceive weaker ones. It is tempting and fairly easy for the powerful – be they transnational corporations or village money-lenders – to coerce or deceive the weak. Those who live on the margins of survival are so vulnerable that a commitment to refrain from coercing or deceiving them demands much more than non-interference and routine bureaucratic and commercial good practice. What looks outwardly like open bargaining and negotiation between parties with unequal power can mask deception or coercion. The first great advantage of approaching issues of justice by way of an account of obligations is that we see more readily that general principles of justice make different demands in different contexts and that just action and policies often demand more than non-interference.

Obligations and Needs

A second great advantage of approaching questions of poverty and hunger by way of a theory of obligations is that we are not restricted to considering those perfect obligations that correspond to human rights. The universalizing construction can also be used to construct principles of imperfect obligation; specifically, the construction can consider human needs.

Human agents are not the abstract rational agents so beloved of social and political science. They are (as advocates of welfare rights emphasize) embodied rational beings whose rationality and agency only develop and survive in adequate material and social conditions. Adequate social conditions themselves collapse without adequate material conditions. Wherever there is endemic hunger, and the poor health and raised death rates that hunger brings, we know that the material conditions necessary for human agency to grow and survive are fragile and failing. If we are to act only on principles that can be acted on by all, we must then do more than refrain from deceit and coercion. Even scrupulous and sensitive adherence to these principles of justice and their appropriate application cannot guarantee that we act on shared standards where some find their very capacities to act threatened. Because human beings are vulnerable and needy, a commitment to act on principles that can be shared by all has to include a commitment to develop capacities to act and to assist those whose capacities to act are insufficient or faltering. It is a matter of obligation to refrain from making a principle of neglect of human potential or of denying the help needed for agency to survive.

Neither developing human potential nor offering needed help can be a matter of perfect obligation for the standard reason that neither is the sort of policy that we can enact completely. We cannot develop all the potential of all human beings; indeed, we cannot even develop all of our own potential (some developments will rule out others) or some potential for everybody. Similarly, we cannot provide all others all the help that they may need in all circumstances if they are to remain agents. Both development of potential and help to those who need it must be selective; neither can be more than a matter of imperfect obligation. Nevertheless, imperfect obligations are obligations; they are not optional forms of self-expression or heroic action that exceeds all obligation.

When we look at the vast scale of human hunger and misery, we may feel that principles of imperfect obligation are just not enough. Surely, we may feel, those who try to establish welfare rights are on the right track. For they try to show that the poor have rights to have their needs met. If welfare rights could be established, they would provide more complete reasons for action to end hunger than principles of imperfect obligation provide. However, if welfare rights cannot be determined, we have good reason to look at the framework of obligations within which rights have a place, but not the whole place. Principles of imperfect obligation are not a trivial matter. They offer not a complete account of what is owed, but an addition to an account of perfect obligations. Helping others and developing human potential are not *substitutes for* but *supplements to* just action. If we are to meet our obligations, we must act to help develop human potential as well as to meet human needs.

We may find courage for these tasks if we realize that our obligation is to do something, not to do everything. For doing something lies within our powers, while doing everything does not. Those of us who are less vulnerable, who hold offices in institutions that have some power, and who are citizens of nations that are not powerless or highly vulnerable may find that quite a lot lies within our powers. We may also find it liberating to think in terms of an account of human obligations that is congruent with the older currents of Western religion and tradition and does not demand that we divide our ethical life into separate public and private spheres and govern them by conflicting principles.

NOTES

1 For various utilitarian views on world hunger, see Singer, Peter (1972) 'Famine, affluence, and morality', *Philosophy and Public Affairs* 1, 229–43; Jackson, Tony

(1982) *Against the Grain*, Oxford, Oxfam; Hardin, Garrett (1974) 'Lifeboat ethics: the case against helping the poor', *Psychology Today*, 8, 38–43 and 123–6. I have discussed these disagreements among utilitarians and other difficulties with ethical reasoning about world hunger in O'Neill, O. (1986) *Faces of Hunger: an essay on poverty, development and justice*, London, George Allen & Unwin.

2 See Dworkin, Ronald (1978) 'Liberalism', in Stuart Hampshire (ed.) *Public and Private Morality*, Cambridge, Cambridge University Press, pp. 113–43. The theme is most deeply explored in MacIntyre, Alasdair (1981) *After Virtue: a study in moral theory*, London, Duckworth.

3 The label is an ill-chosen one because the term 'welfare' has been put to various uses, including (especially in the United States) that of indicating goods and services to which people are *not* entitled. For those who take the term to mean something like 'handout' or 'undeserved benefit', the thought that there could be welfare rights must appear puzzling indeed. This, however, is no more than one of those unhappy historical accidents that happen to quite respectable words. In any case, the claim that there are rights to have basic needs met cannot be rejected by calling such rights welfare rights and then pointing out that the very idea of a welfare right is paradoxical if one assumes a certain interpretation of 'welfare'.

4 The origins of the construction are to be found in the writings of Jean-Jacques Rousseau and Immanuel Kant; it is inserted into rather different, liberal (but non-libertarian) contexts by J. S. Mill and recently by John Rawls and used in a wide variety of ways by contemporary libertarian writers.

5 See, for example, Shue, Henry (1980) *Basic Rights: subsistence, affluence and U. S. foreign policy*, Princeton, NJ, Princeton University Press; Gewirth, Alan (1982) 'Starvation and human rights', in his *Human Rights: essays on justification and application*, Chicago, University of Chicago Press. Gewirth offers reasons why those who take themselves to be agents must hold that they, and so others, have some rights.

6 See Shue, *Basic Rights*.

7 For further clarification of some problems with universalizing constructions, see O'Neill, *Faces of Hunger* and (1989) *Construction of Reason: explorations of Kant's practical philosophy*, Cambridge, Cambridge University Press.

Index

Note: '*n*' after a page reference denotes the number of a note on that page.